JN334459

Quick Tips on
Colonoscopy
Techniques

Edited by Masahiro Igarashi & Shinji Tanaka

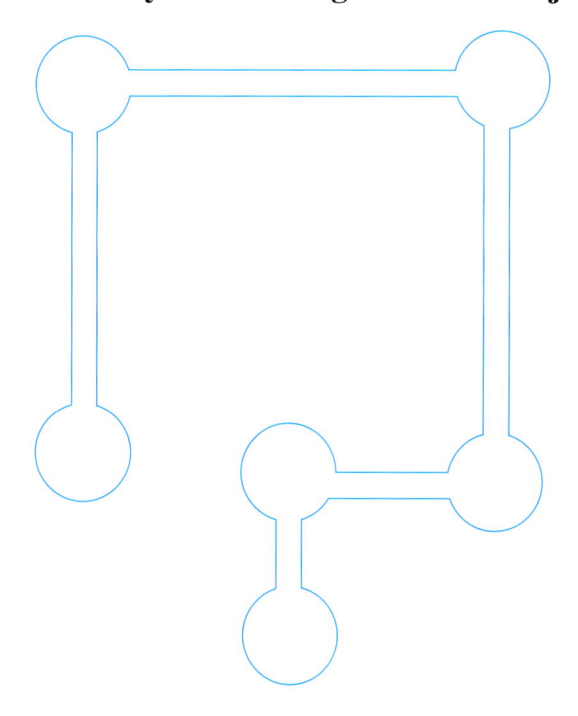

Nihon Medical Center

Quick Tips on Colonoscopy Techniques
Edited by Masahiro Igarashi & Shinji Tanaka

Copyright © 2014 by Nihon Medical Center, Inc.
1-64 Kanda-jinbo-cho, Chiyoda-ku, Tokyo 101-0051, Japan

All rights reserved.
Any reproduction or other unauthorized use of the material or images herein is prohibited without the prior permission of the publisher.

Japanese edition published in Tokyo in 2004 by Nihon Medical Center, Inc.

ISBN: 978-4-88875-270-1

Quick Tips on Colonoscopy Techniques

ワンポイントアドバイス大腸内視鏡検査法〔英語版〕

2014 年 9 月 5 日　第 1 版 1 刷発行

編　集	五十嵐正広／田中　信治
発行者	増永　和也
発行所	株式会社日本メディカルセンター
	東京都千代田区神田神保町 1-64（神保町協和ビル）
	〒101-0051　TEL 03(3291)3901 ㈹
印刷所	シナノ印刷株式会社

ISBN978-4-88875-270-1
©2014　乱丁・落丁は，お取り替えいたします．

本書の複写にかかる複製，上映，譲渡，公衆送信（送信可能化を含む）の各権利は株式会社日本メディカルセンターが管理の委託を受けています．

|JCOPY| <㈳出版者著作権管理機構 委託出版物>

本書の無断複写は著作権法上での例外を除き禁じられています．複写される場合は，そのつど事前に，㈳出版者著作権管理機構（電話 03-3513-6969，FAX03-3513-6979，e-mail：info@jcopy.or.jp）の許諾を得てください．

Authors

Toru Mitsushima
Kameda Medical Center Makuhari

Shinji Tanaka
Department of Endoscopy, Hiroshima University Hospital

Hiroyuki Tsukagoshi
Keiyukai Sapporo Hospital

Satoru Tamura
Division of Gastroenterology, Tamura Clinic

Norihiro Hamamoto
Hamamoto Clinic

Takahisa Matsuda
Endoscopy Division, National Cancer Center Hospital

Masao Ando
Kanagami Hospital

Eisai Cho
Digestive Disease Center, Rakuwakai Otowa Hospital

Hiro-o Yamano
Department of Gastroenterology, Akita Red Cross Hospital

Yuji Inoue
Institute of Gastroenterology, Tokyo Women's Medical University

Sumio Tsuda
Okayama Medical Association, Medical Center

Masahiro Igarashi
Endoscopy Division, Cancer Institute Hospital, Japanese Foundation For Cancer Research

Osamu Tsuruta
Division of Gastroenterology, Department of Medicine, Kurume University School of Medicine / Division of G.I. Endoscopy, Kurume University School of Medicine

Hiroshi Kawano
Division of Gastroenterology, Department of Medicine, Kurume University School of Medicine

Hiroshi Kashida
Department of Gastroenterology and Hepatology, Kinki University Faculty of Medicine

Yusuke Saitoh
Digestive Disease Center, Asahikawa City Hospital

Yasumoto Suzuki
Matsushima Clinic

Recommendation comment

This book is very unique. It is dedicated for the study of colonoscopy insertion – the first critical step in the performance of quality colonoscopy. The various elements particular to colonoscopy insertion are described in detail by a variety of the experts with accompanying illustrative images. The explanations are very useful for students of endoscopy to understand the proper technique of colonoscopy. The book describes in detail the fundamental techniques to handle the colonoscope, position patient and provide abdominal pressure before it then tackles the techniques to advance the colonoscope. Chapters on how to examine the colon, avoid complications in the difficult high-risk cases, and perform image-enhanced endoscopy are shared.

The book can be very useful for the beginner to the advanced level colonoscopist. It provides the technical pearls involved to perform the elegant Japanese colonoscopy short insertion with useful tips on "how to do the different maneuver" and the reasons for the maneuver. We ought to welcome this pioneering effort to making the Japanese endoscopy textbook available worldwide.

July 15, 2014
Roy Soetikno, MD, MS
Clinical Professor of Medicine, Stanford University,
affiliated at the Veterans Affairs Palo Alto Health Care System

Preface to the English Edition

One would expect demand for colonoscopy to be as high outside Japan as it is in Japan. Insertion techniques feature prominently at live demonstrations and always attract a lot of interest from doctors outside Japan. Similarly, when hands-on training courses are offered at international society meetings, there is no shortage of eager applicants. So it would seem that many young doctors outside Japan are just as interested in being able to quickly master colonoscopy insertion techniques as those in Japan.

Yet, oddly enough, few texts on the subject of Japanese colonoscopy insertion techniques have been published in English, which begs the question: how exactly do young doctors overseas learn colonoscopy insertion techniques?

Considering this problem, we thought it would be a good idea to put out an English edition of this book.

What distinguishes this book from others on the subject is that the various elements particular to colonoscopy insertion are broken down into a set of detailed topics, which are then discussed by a variety of experts, each of whom offers tips on the same theme — keeping it as simple as possible.

For the reader, this offers important benefits. First of all, it makes clear that there are multiple opinions on how best to achieve a given goal and different methods for doing so. This gives the reader the opportunity to learn and develop techniques that suit their own style and preferences. Secondly, because this book starts out with basic explanations, it contains a lot of material that will be enormously helpful to colonoscopists who are just beginning their training, as well as those who have already gained a moderate level of experience.

As co-editors-in-chief, it is with great pleasure and the utmost confidence that we recommend this English edition to colonoscopists all over the world. Also, we appreceate the support of Nihon Medical Center (Tokyo, Japan) for the completion of this edition.

April 1, 2013
Shinji Tanaka
Masahiro Igarashi

Preface

In the three decades or so since colonoscopy was first introduced, the tools and instruments used have evolved, with fiberscopes gradually being replaced by videoscopes and HD videoscopes. The scopes themselves have morphed into a wide variety of styles and types — from slim scopes to therapeutic scopes with dual channels, as well as magnification scopes and Variable Stiffness scopes. As the tools have become more sophisticated, so the procedures have become simpler. Insertion, which once was a two-person operation, can now be safely handled by one person.

Nevertheless, progress in insertion techniques has not kept pace with the advances and developments in equipment. Reflecting the difficulties experienced by many endoscopists in mastering colonoscopy techniques, numerous practical guides and feature articles have been published on the subject, while seminars and academic meetings on endoscope insertion methods are well attended.

The simple truth of the matter is that colonoscopy is not something one can master overnight. However, one sure way to improve quickly is to learn and follow the successful methods already established by experts in the field, rather than struggling to master them on your own.

In this book, we have categorized the various topics that characterize colonoscopic examinations, focusing on each topic in detail and including tips from highly experienced endoscopists. This gives readers the opportunity to assess different opinions and methods regarding a single topic and find the solution that best fits their own needs and procedural approach.

Well illustrated with charts and diagrams, this pocket-sized book offers a clear, concise reference that you can carry with you so it is always handy when you need it. We have also included descriptions of basic techniques so it serves as a great introduction to colonoscopy for physicians just getting started in the field, as well as for more experienced practitioners who want to improve their techniques.

April 1, 2004
Masahiro Igarashi, Shinji Tanaka

Contents

1. Amount of Air during Scope Insertion

(1) How to feed the right amount of gas during scope insertion 2

(2) Controlling the amount of air during insertion using the technique "by shortening the colonic fold through bending" 4

1. Amount of air — an especially important factor in colonoscopic insertion / 4
2. Minimizing the amount of air fed during insertion / 4
3. Some tips on hand compression / 5

(3) Three misconceptions about insufflated air 6

1. The more air, the more difficult insertion is / 6
2. Endoscopists tend to insufflate a large amount of air without being aware of it / 6
3. The colon does not recover its original shape once air has been fed in it / 7
4. Colonoscopy becomes harder as the amount of insufflation increases / 7

(4) Amount of air — four associated points 8

1. Optimum air amount / 8
2. Scope manipulation / 8
3. Premedication / 9

4. Conditions leading to increase in air amount / 9

(5) Ways to reduce the amount of air in the intestinal tract ... 10
1. Use minimum air until you've passed the SD junction / 10
2. Palpate the abdomen frequently to help prevent excessive insufflation / 10
3. How to reduce air in the intestinal tract / 11

(6) Controlling the amount of air is critical during scope insertion 12
1. Excessive insufflation is strictly prohibited / 12
2. The secret to insertion is to use air suction properly / 12

2. Changing the Patient's Position and Applying Hand Pressure

(1) Changing the patient's position and applying hand pressure during scope insertion 16
1. Changing the patient's position / 16
2. Hand pressure / 17

(2) Patient positioning and hand pressure: Two very effective and frequently used techniques 18
1. Patient positioning / 18
2. Hand pressure / 19

(3) Essential techniques — Patient positioning and hand pressure 20
1. Is the scope new? / 20
2. Degree of force to use in hand pressure / 20

(4) Tips on patient position change and hand pressure 22

1. Patient positions and patient position change / 22

2. Hand pressure / 22

(5) Roles of patient position change and hand pressure in overcoming difficulties and pains 24

1. Patient position change / 24

2. Hand pressure / 25

(6) Effectiveness of patient position change and hand pressure 28

1. Patient position change / 28

2. Hand pressure / 29

(7) Basic hand pressure points 32

(A) Lower abdominal midline / 32

(B) Right lower abdomen / 32

(C) Left lower abdomen / 32

(D) Left hypochondrium / 33

(E) Upper abdominal midline / 33

(F) Right hypochondrium / 33

3. Using a Sliding Tube

(1) Advantages, disadvantages and precautions when using a sliding tube 36

1. Advantages and disadvantages of the use of sliding tube (ST) / 36

2. How to use the ST / 36

3. Precautions when using the ST / 37

(2) Indications for sliding tube 38

1. Is a sliding tube necessary for colonoscopic insertion? / 38
2. Indications for sliding tube in my case / 39

(3) When is the sliding tube applicable? 40

1. When the scope is warped / 40
2. When deaeration is necessary / 41
3. When retrieving polyps / 41

(4) Tips on use of the sliding tube 42

1. Insert slowly while rotating the tube / 42
2. Effective deaeration and warp prevention / 42
3. Determine applicability based on rectal examination and abdominal palpation before insertion / 43
4. Be careful not to snag the intestinal mucosa / 43

(5) Effective use of the sliding tube 44

1. Effective use of sliding tube during insertion / 44
2. Retrieval of large polyp / 45

4. Insertion into the Rectum

(1) Select a scope appropriate to the patient 48

1. Carefully insert the scope from the anus into the rectum / 48
2. Scope insertion technique / 48

(2) Help the patient relax and get the information you need to perform insertion 50

1. What should be done before performing an examination? / 50
2. Manipulate the scope as if swinging it to the left and right, rather

than pushing / 51

(3) Things that should be done before insertion 52

1. Patient posture and arrangement of the light source and monitor / 52

2. Digital anal examination is also important / 52

3. Do not insert the scope yet / 53

4. Now, begin insertion / 53

(4) Start with a rectal examination 54

1. The importance of performing a rectal examination / 54

2. Inserting the scope into the rectum / 54

3. Rotating the scope inside rectum / 55

(5) "Catching the bend" 56

(6) Insertion into the anus, passage through the anal canal and rectum, and observation of these regions 58

1. Patient position / 58

2. Naked-eye observation of the anus and proximity / 58

3. Digital rectal examination / 58

4. Scope insertion / 59

5. Passing the Rs-S Junction

(1) Passing the rectosigmoid junction using knowledge of the location's contours based on three-dimensional anatomy 62

1. Put the patient in the left lateral position to perform insertion and for observation of the rectum / 62

2. The importance of understanding the shape of the colon based on three-dimensional anatomy / 62
3. Using suction rather than unnecessary insufflation / 63
4. The importance of being able to feel any resistance to the scope / 63

(2) Hooking-the-fold technique and rotation factor 64

(3) Effective use of patient position changes and external abdominal compression 66
1. Basic method for passing the S-top / 66
2. Evaluating patient pain / 67

(4) Getting past the Rs-S junction is the key to a successful colonoscopy 68
1. How to hold the scope / 68
2. Maneuvering with minimal air / 69

(5) Passing through the Rs-S junction the right way is the key to success 70
1. The trick is to pull back the scope just before the junction / 70
2. Imagine pulling an oar / 70
3. Do not push your way through the Rs-S junction / 70

(6) Tips on passage through the Rs-S junction 72

(7) The trick is to reduce the amount of air in the rectum 74

6. Passing the SD Junction

(1) The two basic SD junction passage techniques that need to be mastered 76

1. Passing the SDJ while shortening it from the sigmoid colon / 76
2. Passing the SDJ by pushing the scope from the sigmoid colon / 76

(2) Take the configuration of the sigmoid colon into consideration 78

Pattern A / 78
Pattern B / 78
Pattern C / 79

(3) There are two ways to pass SD: the push method and the pull method 80

1. Push method / 80
2. Pull method / 80

(4) Shortening and stretching techniques for the sigmoid colon 82

1. Sigmoid colon shortening technique / 82
2. Sigmoid colon stretching technique / 82

(5) Methods for passing through the sigmoid colon 84

1. Non-push technique / 84
2. Push technique / 84

(6) The SD junction is the best and most important part for the "straightening and shortening method" of insertion 86

1. Start shortening the sigmoid colon immediately after entering it / 86
2. If the lumen appears on the left of the monitor image / 87
3. Shortening at the S-top / 87
4. If the SD junction is acute / 88

7. Passing the Splenic Flexure

(1) How to deal with problems at the splenic flexure 92
1. Getting from the splenic flexure to the transverse colon / 92
2. If you have trouble passing the splenic flexure / 92

(2) Splenic flexure bending toward the left 93

(3) Tips for smooth passage of the splenic flexure 94
1. Novices have problems with previous methods / 94
2. What to do when passage is difficult / 94

(4) How to achieve smooth insertion into splenic flexure ... 96
1. Before insertion into splenic flexure / 96
2. How to insert the scope into the splenic flexure / 96

(5) Importance of straightening the scope and making the splenic flexure less acute 100
1. Status before splenic flexure passage (straightening of the scope) / 100
2. During splenic flexure passage / 101

(6) What you need to know about splenic flexure passage 104

8. Advancing in the Transverse Colon

(1) After passing through splenic flexure — what next? 108
1. Before advancing into the transverse colon / 108
2. After passing the splenic flexure / 108
3. When the middle section of the transverse colon comes into view / 109

(2) Suction and intestinal tract shortening are also essential in the transverse colon 110
1. Maneuvering in the transverse colon mainly involves counterclockwise rotation / 110
2. Suction brings the hepatic flexure closer / 111

(3) Basic maneuvers and applied techniques 112
1. Basic maneuver / 112
2. If the transverse colon is long / 112
3. If a γ-loop forms in the transverse colon / 112

(4) Key points in passage of transverse colon 114

(5) Tips for advancing the scope in the transverse colon 116
1. Four tips / 116
2. Two basic insertion techniques / 116

(6) The importance of shortening the colon and resolving any loops 118
1. From the splenic flexure to the middle part of the transverse colon / 118
2. From the middle part of transverse colon to the hepatic flexure / 119
3. The key to success is hidden in the regions before the transverse colon / 120

9. Passing the Hepatic Flexure

(1) Remember, "haste makes waste" 122
1. Posture changing (left lateral position) and light manipulation on the right hypochondrium are effective / 122
2. Always keep in mind that "haste makes waste" / 123

(2) Hepatic flexure bending toward the right 124

(3) Hook the flexure with the scope's distal end 126
1. How to approach and pass through the hepatic flexure by pulling and twisting the scope / 126
2. How to approach and pass through the hepatic flexure with pushing of the scope / 127

(4) Taking advantage of the descending phenomenon of the hepatic flexure, together with hand compression on the abdomen and patient position change 128
1. Use of paradoxical movement caused by suction / 128
2. If you have difficulty entering the ascending colon / 128

(5) Using respiratory assistance, patient position change and hand pressure 130
1. Basic maneuver / 130
2. Respiratory assistance and patient position change / 130
3. Hand pressure / 130
4. Sliding tube / 131

(6) Key tips on passing through the hepatic flexure 132

10. From the Cecum to the Terminal Ileum

(1) Indication for terminal ileum insertion and insertion frequency 136
1. Before insertion into the terminal ileum
   (insertion from ascending colon to cecum) / 136
2. Insertion into the terminal ileum / 136

(2) Conditions required for scope insertion into terminal ileum 138
1. Scope insertion into the terminal ileum / 138
2. Scope insertion inside the ileum / 138

(3) Scope insertion from the cecum to the ileum 140
1. Straighten the scope / 140
2. Insert the scope's distal end to the bottom of the cecum / 140
3. Pull the scope so its distal end slides across the lower lip of the ileocecal valve / 140
4. Confirm the ileocecal orifice / 140
5. Confirm the entrance of the terminal ileum / 140
6. Insert the scope into the terminal ileum / 140
7. Insert the scope further toward the oral side of the ileum / 141

(4) Appendix orifice, the terminal point of colonoscopy ... 142

(5) Important tips in the path from cecum to terminal ileum 144

(6) Getting from the cecum to the terminal ileum by preserving the scope's freedom of movement 146

1. Straightening the scope is essential / 146
2. Tips for insertion into the ileocecal valve orifice / 146

11. How to Deal with Cases Where Insertion Is Difficult

1) Postoperative Adhesion

(1) Never use force to manipulate the scope 148
1. Regions where postoperative adhesion occurs frequently / 148
2. Postoperative adhesions in the sigmoid colon / 148
3. Postoperative adhesions in the transverse colon / 149
4. Cautions for postoperative adhesion cases / 149

(2) Carefully pass each fold, using as little air as possible 150
1. Use a slim scope for post-gynecological cancer removal or post-C-section cases / 150
2. Post-colectomy cases / 151
3. Post-gastrectomy or post-cholecystectomy cases / 151

(3) Always assume that an adhesion may be present before insertion 152
1. Air suction and repeated shortening little by little are important / 152
2. Is hand pressure useful? / 152
3. Is patient posture change useful? / 153
4. What kind of scope should be used? / 153
5. There is no quick solution for adhesion cases / 153
6. Do not blame everything on adhesions / 153

(4) Areas where insertion is difficult vary depending on whether and where the patient has undergone surgery 154

1. After gynecological surgery / 154
2. After gastrectomy / 154
3. After cholecystectomy / 155

(5) Tips for insertion in postoperative adhesion cases 156

(6) Take a surgical history in the pre-procedure interview 158

2) Dolichocolon (Sigmoid Colon, Transverse Colon)

(1) Dolichocolon and air insufflation 160
1. Misunderstanding on hooking the fold / 160
2. If the colon is stretched to the limit / 160
3. Transverse colon / 161

(2) Measures to be taken before and after sigmoid colon insertion 162
1. What is dolichocolon? / 162
2. Steps to take before insertion into the sigmoid colon / 162
3. Steps to take after sigmoid colon insertion / 163

(3) How to handle the case of dolichocolon (long colon) 164
1. Things you can do to deal with dolichosigmoid / 164
2. Things you can do to deal with dolichotransversum / 165

(4) Countermeasures against dolichosigmoid 166
1. If double loops form / 166
2. If a large loop has formed / 167

(5) Ways to deal with dolichocolon cases 170
1. Dolichosigmoid / 170
2. Dolichotransverse / 171

3) Other

(1) Advanced obesity cases 174
1. What insertion difficulties can advanced obesity cause? / 174
2. Maneuvering the scope when using the push technique / 174
3. Hand pressure and patient position change / 174
4. Other measures / 175

(2) Patients undergoing pelvic radiation, patients with multiple sigmoid diverticula, thin women, elderly patients and patients with bloody stools 176
1. Use a slim scope in cases that have undergone pelvic radiation or with multiple sigmoid diverticula / 176
2. A slim scope is also useful with thin women and elderly patients / 177
3. Emergency colonoscopy for bloody stool / 177

(3) Dealing with adhesions, patients whose position cannot be changed, transverse colon loops, sigmoid colon volvulus and melena 178
1. Cases with adhesion / 178
2. Cases where position change is not possible / 178
3. Cases with loop in the transverse colon / 178
4. Cases with sigmoid colon volvulus / 179
5. Cases with melena

12. Examining Elderly Patients (80 or Older)

(1) Caution is required for insertion in elderly patients 182
1. Causes of insertion difficulties in elderly patients (80 or older) / 182
2. Countermeasures against causes of insertion difficulties / 183

(2) Watch out for any changes in vital signs 186
1. Precautions when examining elderly patients (80 or older) / 186
2. Preparation / 186
3. Sedation / 186
4. Insertion method / 187
5. Recovery / 187

(3) The importance of avoiding risks and knowing when to stop 188
1. Preparation / 188
2. Sedation / 188
3. Insertion method / 189
4. Knowing when to stop / 189

(4) Elderly patients usually have more fragile colons 190
1. Recognize the correct physical age of each patient / 190
2. Be sure to obtain accurate clinical and medication histories / 190
3. Colonoscopy precautions / 191

(5) Key points when examining patients aged 80 or older 192

13. Preventing Perforation during Insertion

(1) Do not use force to manipulate the scope 196
1. The cause of perforation during insertion / 196
2. Unnecessary scope manipulation / 196
3. Prevention of perforation during insertion / 197

(2) Always perform insertion carefully and be prepared to discontinue the procedure before completion 198
1. Causes of perforation / 198
2. If insertion is difficult / 199

(3) The importance of identifying high-risk cases 200
1. Make sure to conduct a full interview and consultation before the examination / 200
2. Observe the basic rules of insertion / 201
3. Always be prepared to discontinue the procedure if necessary / 201

(4) Avoid applying excessive force to the colon wall 202
1. Causes of perforation during scope insertion / 202
2. How to avoid applying direct force to the colon wall / 202
3. How to avoid applying indirect force to the colon wall / 203

(5) Situations where perforation can occur and how to avoid them 204
1. When scope control is difficult / 204
2. When the image shown during contact with the mucosa (completely red) cannot be moved / 204
3. When removing the loop / 204
4. When the patient complains of pain after the procedure / 205

5. Things to keep in mind in order to avoid perforation / 205

6. Cautions on use of sedative and analgesic / 205

(6) When caution is required during insertion 206

1. Perforation in the vicinity of SD junction / 206

2. Example of multiple sigmoid diverticulums / 206

3. Adhesion / 207

14. Observation Tips

(1) When is the best time for observation? 210

1. During insertion or during withdrawal? / 210

2. Observation method / 210

3. Residual fluids and bubbles / 211

4. Insufflation and deaeration / 211

(2) Observation by withdrawing the scope a little at a time 212

1. Use an anticholinergic agent for observation / 212

2. Use retroflexed observation in the right-side colon / 212

3. Put the region to be observed in the highest position / 212

4. Observe the inner sides of the bends carefully / 213

5. Observe the sigmoid colon by re-inserting scope / 213

6. Use retroflexed observation in the vicinity of the anus / 213

7. Use dyes as required / 213

(3) Always pay attention to superficial elevated type and depressed type lesions 214

1. Viewing without noticing / 214

2. Pay attention to slight differences in color tone and gloss / 214

3. Insufflation does not always make lesions more noticeable / 214
4. Patient posture change is often useful / 215
5. Dye spraying is essential / 215

(4) How to avoid missing lesions in blind spots 216
1. During insertion / 216
2. During withdrawal / 216
3. Varying the amount of air / 217
4. Easily missed lesions / 217

(5) Tips on detection and diagnosis 220
1. Tips on detection / 220
2. Tips on diagnosis / 221

(6) Tips on accurate qualitative diagnosis using standard colonoscopic observation 224
1. Discard preconceived ideas when screening / 224
2. Tips on standard colonoscopic observation of a localized lesion / 224
3. Observation using dye spraying / 225
4. Tips on washing the lesion / 225

(7) Important points to keep in mind during observation 226

15. Retroflexed Observation in the Rectum

(1) Rectal observation is a must 230
1. Why retroflexed observation in the rectum is necessary / 230
2. The key to mastering colonoscopy is the ileocecal valve insertion method / 231

(2) Observation without dead angles 232
 1. Observing the anterior wall during withdrawal / 232
 2. Retroflexed observation technique / 232
 3. Observation method / 232

(3) The purpose of retroflexed observation and some points to remember 234
 1. Retroflexion method / 234
 2. Retroflexed observation / 234
 3. Danger of injury / 235

(4) Do not take it easy during observation of the rectum 236
 1. Why so many lesions are missed in the rectum / 236
 2. Retroflex observation / 236
 3. Precautions for retroflexion / 237
 4. Other techniques useful for observing the rectum / 237

(5) Eliminating blind spots in rectal observation by retroflexing the scope 238
 1. Retroflexion in the rectum / 238
 2. Retroflexed observation / 238

16. Dye Spraying
 (1) Dye spraying, safety of dyes 242

 (2) Reasons for dye spraying and how to do it 244
 1. Chromoendoscopy in the colon and rectum / 244
 2. Dye-spraying procedure / 244

3. Points to heed when spraying the dye / 245

(3) Contrasting technique 246
1. Washing the lesion and surrounding area / 246
2. Dye spraying / 246

(4) Contrast method and staining method 248
1. Contrast method / 248
2. Staining method / 248
3. Appropriate applications for each method / 249

(5) Tips on dye spraying and observation 250
1. Contrast method / 250
2. Staining method / 251

(6) How to wash lesions and spray dyes 252
1. First, wash away mucus and stool liquid attached to the surface of the lesion / 252
2. Tips on washing the lesion / 252
3. Contrast method using indigo carmine / 254
4. Staining method using crystal violet / 254

om
1. Amount of Air during Scope Insertion

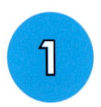

1 How to feed the right amount of gas during scope insertion

Toru Mitsushima

Just about any endoscopist will tell you that if you insufflate too much gas, it gets more difficult to move the scope forward smoothly. The pitfall is that in order to view the lumen on the proximal side, many novices to endoscopy tend to insufflate too much gas to advance the scope.

One way to overcome this problem is to inject about 300 ml of barium sulfate into the rectum and send it toward the proximal-side colon without insufflating gas, that is, by taking advantage of its own weight while changing the patient's position, the barium can reach the ascending colon relatively smoothly without forming complicated bends. This can be clearly observed under fluoroscopy.

As long as only barium is injected without insufflation, no acute bends will form — even in that part of the intestinal canal between the sigmoid colon and the descending colon, which is normally considered the most difficult in colonoscopy (**Fig. 1-1-1**). However, once gas is insufflated to obtain a double-contrast image, the condition changes completely. The insufflation not only pushes out the pliable colon wall in the short-axis direction, enlarging the diameter of the colon, but also extends the intestinal wall in the long-axis direction, producing acute, complicated bends (**Fig. 1-1-2**: double-contrast image of the same patient in the supine position as in Fig. 1-1-1).

When scope insertion proves difficult during colonoscopy, the first thing the endoscopist should consider is the possibility that excessive insufflation may have produced the situation shown in Fig. 1-1-2. This means that, if we stick to the basic colonoscopic insertion technique of advancing the scope while trying to avoid stretching the intestinal tract and smoothing out any bends, then we recommend that the amount of gas insufflated during scope insertion be kept to an absolute minimum.

Now, some are of the opinion that the gas switch on the light source should be set to OFF when the scope is inserted, so that there is no chance of gas insufflation. However, I consider this a bit extreme. If there is too little gas in the intestinal tract, it becomes difficult to locate the proximal side of the lumen, thus increasing the difficulty of insertion. In addition, gas is also necessary to facilitate careful observation of the mucosal surface during scope insertion.

In particular, in those parts of the intestinal tract characterized by a complex series of bends, such as the section from the rectosigmoid colon to the sigmoid colon and descending colon, very delicate maneuvering is required, which involves pushing the gas button once to dilate the proximal-side lumen for checking, then immediately pushing the suction button to deaerate and pass the bend.

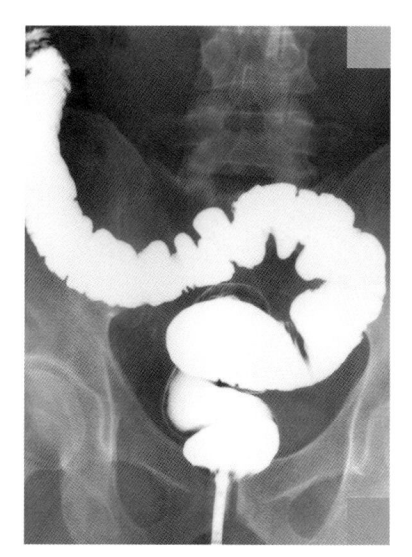

Fig. 1-1-1 Barium enem image without gas insufflation

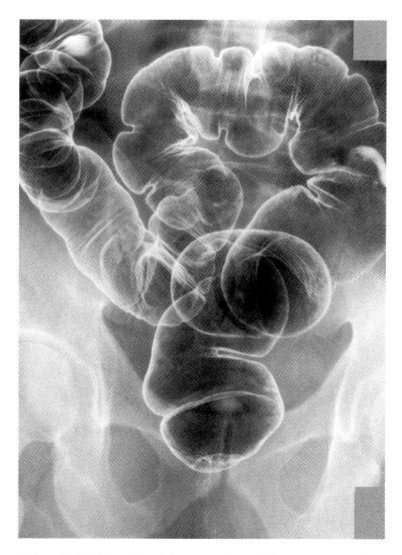

Fig. 1-1-2 Double-contrast image of the same patient in the supine position as in Fig. 1-1-1

② Controlling the amount of air during insertion using the technique "by shortening the colonic fold through bending"

Shinji Tanaka

1. Amount of air — an especially important factor in colonoscopic insertion

One of the keys to mastering colonoscopic insertion is to learn how to properly manage the amount of air insufflated during a procedure. Those endoscopists who have a low success rate when attempting "to shorten the colonic fold through bending", despite being skilled at maneuvering the scope, tend to insufflate too much air during insertion. Even while not intending to insufflate air, their fingers inadvertently touch the air button and activate insufflation.

If endoscopists base their procedure on the assumption that a sufficient field of view must first be obtained in the intestinal lumen, and then advancing past the colonic bends by pushing, and then shortening the colon, they will never be able to advance beyond a certain stage.

2. Minimizing the amount of air fed during insertion

Excessive insufflation during insertion from the rectum to the sigmoid colon makes it pretty much impossible to successfully continue a procedure. Minimizing the amount of insufflation during insertion in order to make the bends gradual without stretching the intestinal tract is one of the most critical points in performing successful colonoscopy. In other words, it is important to remember that the scope should be advanced using suction to pull in the intestinal bends and fold them in the form like a bellows by turning or pulling back the scope rather than pushing it.

Using simple suction to reduce air in the intestinal tract makes it possible to insert the scope more naturally and to more easily manipulate it. This is particularly important to enable linear insertion without pushing the top of the sigmoid colon upwards. The procedure sometimes has to be done blind when pulling back in the position of the top of the sigmoid colon.

3. Some tips on hand compression

If it looks like the top of the sigmoid colon is going to be pushed upwards despite careful manipulation, this can often be avoided by hand compresion on the suprapubic region. This should be done using the fingertips or fists (pointed application), rather than the palms. It is usually done with the patient in the left lateral position, but can also be done with the patient in the supine position. Changing the position would move the air inside the intestinal tract, thereby making the top of the sigmoid colon more gradual and facilitating rotary insertion of the scope.

Hand compression on the abdomen in the supine position is also very effective. If extension of the top of the sigmoid colon cannot be avoided even when using this method, advance the scope as far as the SD junction (by about 50 cm at maximum), while applying hand compresion to prevent the intestinal tract from extending excessively and then try to shorten the inserted length of the scope. If the scope can be inserted smoothly along the intestinal axis with as little air as possible, the patient will feel little if any pain. Typically, when insertion is problematic, the amount of air that is insufflated tends to increase, when what actually is necessary is to suction the air in order to reduce the air in the intestinal tract.

By deliberately using less insufflation than you would normally use during insertion and by applying hand compression on the abdomen or changing the patient's position as required, you will be able to improve the success rate "to shorten the colonic fold through bending".

③ Three misconceptions about insufflated air

Hiroyuki Tsukagoshi

1. The more air, the more difficult insertion is
There are two factors that make colonoscopic insertion difficult. One is when the scope has to be passed through a sharp curve and the second is when the scope warps, making it impossible to transmit force even when the scope is pushed. Everyone who performs colonoscopy knows how important it is to minimize the amount of air insufflated. The more the air increases, the more difficult insertion becomes.

However, as most endoscopists who are starting out in colonoscopy usually have a fair amount of experience with upper GI cases, they are used to creating a field of view by insufflating air during insertion. Even though they know that the air should be reduced in colonoscopy and are confident that they are using enough suction, they still tend to insufflate too much air in the colon.

In my experience, there are three main reasons for this.

2. Endoscopists tend to insufflate a large amount of air without being aware of it
First, despite the fact that many endoscopists are convinced that they insufflate a small amount of air in the relatively easy sections of the colon, and perform suction as required to reduce air in the difficult sections, they actually tend to feed a large amount of air in order to ensure the field of view, without being aware that they are doing so.

Specifically, while the amount of insufflation actually required until the splenic flexure is reached is 50 to 100 ml, many endoscopists insufflate 1,000 to 2,000 ml of air. It is important for endoscopists to recognize that their insertion methods typically involve the unconscious insufflation of a large amount of air.

3. The colon does not recover its original shape once air has been fed in it

The second misconception is that too much insufflation can always be offset by performing suction. In fact, once the colon has been stretched by feeding air into it, the original shape of the colon cannot be recovered. Moreover, suction can only deaerate the region in proximity to the tip of the scope, not those areas distant from the scope tip.

4. Colonoscopy becomes harder as the amount of insufflation increases

The third misconception is the belief that the cecum of 90% of patients can be reached quickly regardless of the insertion technique, provided that the endoscopist is experienced, and that insertion can be completed more quickly by insufflating air to ensure the field of view. Many endoscopists also tend to think that the insertion difficulties with the other 10% of patients are due to adhesion or the like, and that some level of discomfort is unavoidable during insertion.

While it is true that there are actually cases in which insertion is difficult, there is no doubt that insertion will get more difficult as the amount of insufflation increases. Even though the field of view in more difficult cases is likely to be poorer, it is still necessary to use as little air as possible.

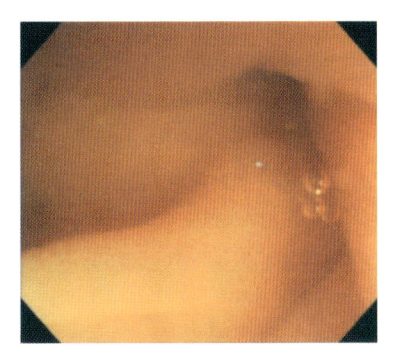

Fig. 1-3-1 Without insufflation: Rs junction

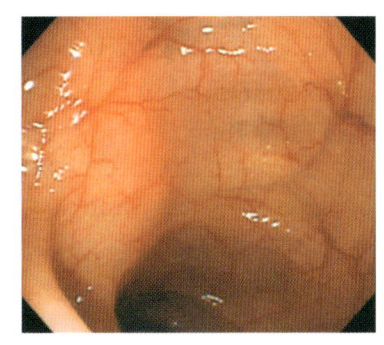

Fig. 1-3-2 With excessive insufflation: Sigmoid colon

④ Amount of air — four associated points

Satoru Tamura

1. Optimum air amount

In order to insert a colonoscope, a certain amount of air must be insufflated to expand the lumen and monitor the direction of the scope. The problem here is that excessive insufflation the bends of intestinal tract more acute and makes insertion harder. When dilated by air, the intestinal bends take on a valve-like shape. This makes it more difficult to perform the shortening maneuver by hooking the scope tip to the oral side, forcing the endoscopist to attempt insertion by relying on the push operation, which causes pain to the patient.

To avoid this, the amount of air should be reduced to a level that is just enough to check the contour of the colon. The point here is that an intestinal tract that becomes somewhat like a drainage tile due to excessive air insufflation should be deaerated by early suction to perform insertion.

2. Scope manipulation

We often see endoscopists (novices, in particular) continue insufflation during manipulation of the scope, without being aware that they are doing so. One way to prevent this is to use the left hand properly. Those who are accustomed to the manipulation of upper GI scopes perform examinations by hooking the index and middle fingers permanently on two buttons — the suction and air/water buttons.

With colonoscopy, however, only a single finger — the index finger — should be used, alternating between the suction and air/water buttons as required, while holding the scope with the middle, ring and little fingers.

3. Premedication

Administration of an antispasmodic is necessary to avoid excessive insufflation. In an intestinal tract accompanied with strong peristalsis, endoscopists frequently tend to unconsciously increase insufflation in order to check the contour of the lumen.

4. Conditions leading to increase in air amount

The most unfavorable patient condition is the spastic colon. In an intestinal tract with strong spasms, repeated waves of peristalses make it hard to confirm the conditions inside the lumen. To check the contour, insufflation is increased. However, this only expands the lumen temporarily. As the amount of air increases, conditions become even more difficult and more painful for the patient.

The best way to cope with this is to have patience, waiting for the peristalses to subside and then inserting the scope a little deeper. Once the sigmoid colon has been passed and the descending colon is entered, the scope can be inserted deeply without worrying about peristalses. The key, then, to getting past the sigmoid colon, is patience.

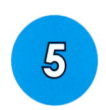

⑤ Ways to reduce the amount of air in the intestinal tract

Norihiro Hamamoto

1. Use minimum air until you've passed the SD junction

Beginners are often so concerned with getting past the folds that they have a tendency to insufflate too much air. Needless to say, manipulating the scope with as little air as possible facilitates smooth, painless colonoscopy. Careless insufflation during insertion from the rectum to the sigmoid colon can cause dilation of the sigmoid colon, making straight insertion extremely difficult when approaching the next lumen from the S-top. A loop will also form, making up to the SD junction more painful for the patient.

Though it is hard to say just how much air is the right amount, we can say that you should only touch the air button momentarily to identify the orientation of the next lumen, which should always be kept in the collapsed status. When the curves of the folds are tensed, that means there is too much air. If it is difficult to estimate the orientation of the intestinal tract, the trick is to advance the scope by referring to the directions of the folds and the flow of irrigation water, while keeping the scope distal end as close as possible to the intestinal mucosa (to the point just before the field of view fills up with an indiscernible red image).

2. Palpate the abdomen frequently to help prevent excessive insufflation

Once blown in, air cannot be suctioned easily. In practice, air has often penetrated deeper regions even when the intestinal tract looks collapsed on the monitor screen.

It is also important to identify the amount of air insufflated in the colon. If you feel you have insufflated too much air, try performing frequent palpations of the abdomen to identify how much air has been insufflated.

This means you will have to check the original condition of the abdomen before scope insertion.

3. How to reduce air in the intestinal tract

To reduce the air already in the tract or that was insufflated during insertion before approaching the next lumen, catch a fold in the upward direction, pull it back slightly, and activate suction a little at a time. Repeat this procedure a few more times. This will eliminate intestinal tract traction and may open the view to the next lumen.

This technique is also effective when advancing through the lumen with downward manipulation during insertion from the S-top to the sigmoid colon. Nevertheless, with this technique, care is required not to absorb the mucosa in the suction outlet on the scope tip.

Deaeration methods other than suction include:
① asking the patient to try to break wind from the anus;
② inserting a sliding tube.

Method ① is not easy because the scope is being inserted into the anus, but is sometimes effective when straightening the scope formed into a loop. If the scope is inserted into the proximity of the splenic flexure of a patient who has a long sigmoid colon, method ② is effective for removing air in the left side of the colon. However, this method requires care because it presents a risk of accidentally damaging the mucosa and perforating it if the scope is not straight.

⑥ Controlling the amount of air is critical during scope insertion

Takahisa Matsuda

1. Excessive insufflation is strictly prohibited

Since most endoscopists start out upper GI endoscopy, they get into the habit of keeping a finger on the air button, something that carries over into colonoscopy, especially with novices. In upper GI endoscopy, the best way to control the amount of air is simply to insufflate to the point just before the patient starts to belch.

During colonoscopy, on the other hand, the best way to control the air and residual fluid in the intestinal tract is through suctioning. Excessive insufflation in the colon makes it difficult to insert the scope "by shortening the colonic fold through bending". When the intestinal tract is stretched by insufflation, the shortening of the intestinal tract at the S-top (at about 20 cm AV), which is encountered immediately after the start of examination, is more difficult to get past because it forms an acute bend. Too much air can also increase the patient's discomfort during the shortening manipulation of the region. Therefore, excessive insufflation must be avoided until the sigmoid colon is passed.

2. The secret to insertion is to use air suction properly

The secret to smooth insertion is to effectively control the amount of air in the intestinal tract by means of suction. For example, a patient with a relatively long sigmoid colon often has the S-top at a higher position than usual (high S-top: **Fig. 1-6-1**). In this case, the scope tip should reach the acute bend in the upper right direction (this is the S-top) at a longer-than-usual distance. At this time, utilizing the suction properly makes it possible to lower the S-top and cause it to approach the scope's distal end. Then, by rotating the scope clockwise, it can be advanced past the S-top without stretching it. The thing to remember here is that the shortening manipulation becomes difficult if the scope is inserted by pushing until it reaches the distant S-top position.

This applies not only to the S-top, but also to insertion from the transverse colon (mid-T) across the hepatic flexure. The scope should not be inserted into the final curve (hepatic flexure) by pushing. Instead, suction the air at a position past the mid-T so that the hepatic flexure approaches the scope, and then insert the scope as if dropping it into the ascending colon, while rotating clockwise. Doing it this way avoids any patient discomfort.

In short, scope insertion with the technique "by shortening the colonic fold through bending" basically involves suctioning air and residual fluid in the intestinal tract properly (without suctioning the mucosa), and proximally pulling in the intestinal tract in front and contracting it by folding.

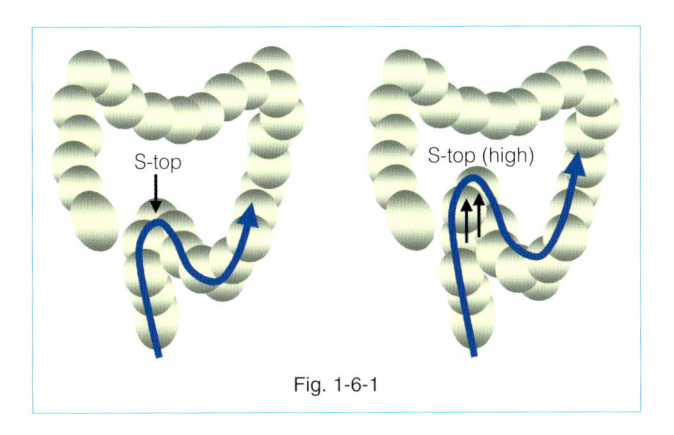

Fig. 1-6-1

2. Changing the Patient's Position and Applying Hand Pressure

1 Changing the patient's position and applying hand pressure during scope insertion

Toru Mitsushima

When it is difficult to advance the scope in colonoscopy, two techniques for dealing with are changing the patient's position and applying hand pressures.

1. Changing the patient's position

As I use a slim colonoscope that can easily get bent out of shape, I usually change position of the patient position at a relatively early stage of procedure. For scope insertion from the anus to the oral side of rectum (Ra), I put the patient in the left lateral position, frequently changing the patient to the supine position for insertion through the rectum and sigmoid colon section (Rs). This prevents excessive stretching of the intestinal tract between the Rs and the sigmoid colon and minimizes the patient's discomfort.

In the section from the sigmoid colon and descending colon flexure (SD flexure), passing the splenic flexure (SF) and finally reaching the ascending colon and cecum, I advance the scope almost exclusively with the patient in the supine position. This takes advantage of gravity to reduce the deflection of the sigmoid colon toward the abdominal side, which interferes with smooth forward movement of the scope.

If bends in the colon make it difficult to advance the scope from the descending colon to the SF section, placing the patient in the right lateral position can often be effective. In cases where it is difficult to advance the scope across the hepatic flexure (HF) in the supine position due to residual stool, putting the patient in the left or right lateral position will usually solve the problem.

2. Hand pressure

The illustrations below show the three hand pressure patterns I use most often (**Figs. 2-1-1a, b, c**).

The method in Fig. 2-1-1a is applied when the scope has formed a loop in the sigmoid colon and cannot be advanced smoothly because the scope is bent toward the cranial and abdominal sides. This method is often very helpful regardless of whether the scope's distal end is located in the sigmoid colon, descending colon or transverse colon.

The method in Fig. 2-1-1b is applicable to cases in which the sigmoid colon is long and the SD flexure forms a sharp bend. It is effective when the scope cannot be advanced to the oral side of the descending colon, even though the scope's distal end has already passed the SD flexure and the loop has been released.

The method in Fig. 2-1-1c is useful when the scope has been bent by the sagging of the transverse colon and cannot be moved past the HF. This is the hand pressure method I use most frequently with a slim scope.

It is important to be careful when applying hand pressure because if it is applied too early, for example in the sigmoid colon, the scope could get twisted unnaturally, making it difficult to maneuver in the deep part of the rectum. Try to avoid using hand pressure until the scope's distal end reaches the HF section, advancing the scope to that point by relying only on patient position changes whenever possible.

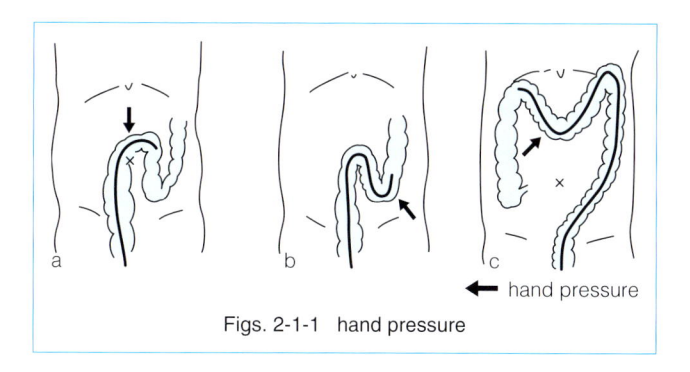

Figs. 2-1-1 hand pressure

② Patient positioning and hand pressure: Two very effective and frequently used techniques

Masao Ando

1. Patient positioning

1) During insertion

Start insertion with the patient in the left lateral position and change to the supine position once you get past the rectosigmoid (Rs). Together with the application of hand pressure, this will help to significantly shorten the sigmoid colon. Keep the patient in the supine position until the scope reaches the splenic flexure. With female patients, the presence of the uterus may make the left lateral position more effective. Temporarily switching to the right lateral position may also be effective if there is any difficulty shortenings the sigmoid colon.

When advancing the scope downward from the splenic flexure to the transverse colon, the right lateral position is the most effective. This position also helps reduce patient discomfort. Having the patient take deep breaths at optimum times can also be helpful.

When the scope enters the transverse colon, place the patient back in the supine position.

If you have any difficulty getting past the hepatic flexure, you may find it helpful to put the patient in the right lateral position and perform suction as required. If it is difficult to advance the scope downward to the ascending colon, use the supine position again. Sometimes the optimum instant for advancing the scope can occur while changing to the supine position.

If it is impossible to advance the scope, either by pushing or pulling, while the cecum is in view, switch immediately to the right lateral positions.

2) During observation

Use the supine position for withdrawal. As one would in an enema examination, keep in mind the relationship between the residual fluids and the dilation of intestinal tract while changing the patient's position. In the ascending colon, you can use both the supine and left lateral positions.

A slightly right lateral position is recommended from the middle of the transverse colon. Usually it is sufficient to have the patient lift the left hip slightly. This can dilate the intestinal tract without using excessive air and reduce patient discomfort.

At the sigmoid colon, return the patient to the supine position. Complete the examination with retroflexed observation in the left lateral position.

The above is the routine pattern of the present author. The readers can naturally apply their own contrivances according to each case.

2. Hand pressure

This technique has two different purposes, and should be regarded as a completely different procedure depending on the purpose. One purpose is to attenuate sagging of the intestinal tract and the other is to allow the scope to pass the next folds.

Prevention of sagging includes the following cases:
1) hand pressure from the left inferior abdomen toward the umbilicus in case of difficulty in passing the SD section;
2) clipping of the section between the left abdomen and right inferior abdomen for preventing sagging of the S section;
3) prevention of sagging of the transverse colon.

It is important to emphasize that hand pressure is very effective in supporting scope insertion from the sigmoid colon past the SD junction without any stretching the intestinal tract (with "non-push" operation). If it is impossible to pass the final fold by shortening, find the region where the fold comes closest in the image (this is often the suprapubic area) and, while pressing the region gently, pass the fold by rotating the scope ("press & pass" operation). This assumes that deaeration is sufficient and that the scope is basically straightened. Insertion skill will improve dramatically once you get a feel for this technique because it is applicable to insertion in other regions, as well.

③ Essential techniques — Patient positioning and hand pressure

Hiroyuki Tsukagoshi

Patient positioning and hand pressure are essential for successful insertion in colonoscopies. The difficulty of insertion can vary widely from one patient to the next.

The degree of difficulty can be categorized as easy, average and hard. Easy cases permit insertion as far as the cecum in the left lateral position, with neither patient position change nor hand pressure being necessary. With such cases, skilled endoscopists can reach the cecum in 2 or 3 minutes, and even novices only take 10 minutes to reach the cecum.

1. Is the scope new?

In about 50% of average cases, the scope sometimes warps at the splenic flexure. If this happens, the patient must be placed in the supine position and hand pressure applied, if necessary. The frequency of patient repositioning and hand pressure application depends on the type of the scope in use, as well as the degree of difficulty. The frequency decreases when the scope in use is thicker and stiffer, and increases when the scope is slimmer and more flexible. It is also worth noting that scope stiffness varies depending on how old the scope is. The older the scope, the more flexible it becomes.

2. Degree of force to use in hand pressure

Splenic flexure: This section can often be entered easily by simply putting the patient in the supine position. However, with relatively difficult cases, it can be effective to add hand pressure. Hand pressure is performed by an assistant who pushes the umbilical area gently with the palms of their hands. Strong force is not necessary. Using too much force can also tire the assistant, making them less able to perform their tasks efficiently. All the assistant needs to do is straighten their elbows and lean on the patient. What is important is the height of the examination table. As appropriate pressure is impossible to apply if it is too high, it is necessary to adjust the table height or use a footstool.

If it is impossible to advance the scope into the splenic flexure, it may be easier to switch the patient to the right lateral position, but I don't recommend this. Patient repositioning and hand pressure are not necessarily required for advancement in the splenic flexure. The only reason for using them is to save time. Difficulty in advancing in the splenic flexure indicates that there is a problem with the insertion technique. Most of the time, the cause of this problem is too much air, as discussed in Chapter 1.

Hepatic flexure: When it is difficult to advance in the hepatic flexure, it may be helpful to put the patient in the supine position. There is no need to use hand pressure; however, instead, I ask the patient to take deep breaths. If this doesn't do the trick, the quickest, easiest thing to do is push the scope to stretch the transverse colon as far as the pelvis and then hook the scope tip on the ascending colon. It is a waste of time to try advancing the scope straight.

Sigmoid colon: If insertion into the sigmoid colon is impossible due to patient obesity or an adhesion, the only solution is to push the scope. The scope length may become insufficient or hand pressure by two persons may sometimes be required. To determine which location to compress, compress various regions to see which one the sigmoid colon looks closest to in the endoscopic image. In some cases, compression is required to prevent too much bending of the scope or to reduce the volume of the abdomen.

There may be cases where insertion is extremely difficult, though such cases are rare, perhaps as few as one in several hundred. If it is absolutely necessary to observe the deep part of the colon with such a case, the only way is to use the supine position, manipulate the scope mainly by pushing and use hand pressure optimally. Whether or not this succeeds depends on the skill of the person(s) applying the hand pressure.

4 Tips on patient position change and hand pressure

Eisai Cho

1. Patient positions and patient position change

Let's look at the most appropriate patient positions according to the location of the distal end of a scope.

Insertion: The basic patient position is the left lateral position. This is the position in which visual inspection and expansion of the anus, palpation of the rectum and insertion of the scope can be done most smoothly.

Rectum to descending colon: The basic patient position is the left lateral position. The supine position is used when the sigmoid colon or SD junction forms an acute angle or when insertion is not smooth.

Descending colon to ascending colon: The basic patient position is the supine position. In the splenic flexure, changing to the right lateral position sometimes facilitates advancement of the scope into the transverse colon by taking advantage of the scope's own weight. In the hepatic flexure, changing to the left lateral position sometimes facilitates insertion by improving the field of view.

Ascending colon to cecum: The basic patient position is the supine position. If it is difficult to advance the scope in this section, change to the left anterior oblique position to facilitate insertion by taking advantage of the scope's own weight.

Insertion from the rectum to the cecum is sometimes possible while the patient is in the left lateral position, but it can be facilitated by using the basic patient position best suited to each section.

2. Hand pressure

Hand pressure is performed while the inserted part of the scope is shortened and straightened. When the intestinal tract is stretched or looped, compression is less effective due to difficulty in transmitting force. The important thing is to avoid creating abdominal wall tension. This means that compression should not be applied suddenly with a lot of force. It is necessary to apply compression gradually and gently to avoid tension. Hand pressure performed by the patients themselves can sometimes be quite effective.

Descending colon to transverse colon: If it is difficult to advance beyond the descending colon, the scope may be extended and looped in the sigmoid colon.

- S-point (**Fig. 2-4-1**): In general, compress a broad area in the left lower abdomen from the front toward the back. Compressing the sigmoid colon along an oblique line following the scope could stretch the sigmoid colon toward the front. Therefore, it is better to compress a broad area of the left lower abdomen toward the back so that the sigmoid colon is not stretched toward the front. In rare cases, the sigmoid colon is stretched outwards to the left. In this case, apply compression from the outer side of the left abdominal wall toward the inner side.

Transverse colon to ascending colon: If it is difficult to advance from the transverse colon to the hepatic flexure, either the transverse colon or sigmoid colon or both may be stretched.

- T-point (**Fig. 2-4-2**): Compress the center of the upper abdomen from the front toward the upper part of the back to prevent sagging of the transverse colon. If compression of the T-point alone is ineffective, compress the S-point or both of the T- and S-points.

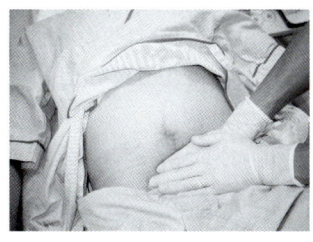

Fig. 2-4-1 Hand pressure on the S-point

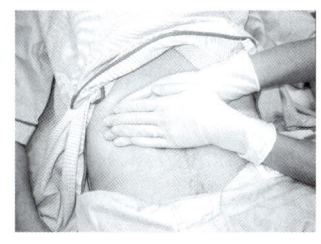

Fig. 2-4-2 Hand pressure on the T-point

⑤ Roles of patient position change and hand pressure in overcoming difficulties and pains
Hiro-o Yamano

Changing the patient's position and applying hand pressure are two of the most effective ways to deal with difficult colonoscope insertion.

1. Patient position change
By changing the patient's position, we can take advantage of the force of gravity to advance the colonoscope. The effects of these changes are summarized below.

1) Change in intestinal tract shape due its own weight
The part of the intestinal tract not attached to the retroperitoneum has a certain degree of mobility even if the mesentery is attached. However, the range of mobility may be limited by the balance between the weight of the intestinal tract and the traction produced by the mesentery.

When the patient position is changed, the entire intestine moves left and right and forward and back, changing the angles of the various bends including the hepatic flexure and splenic flexure, making some more acute angle and some less.

2) Improvement of intestinal lumen by movement of air and fluids inside the intestinal tract
Changing the patient's position causes air and fluids in the intestinal tract to move according to the force of gravity. For instance, when the patient is placed in the right lateral position, the air moves to the left side of the tract opposite to the direction of gravity, dilating the lumen and creating a space. During insertion of colonoscope, this effect makes it easier to clarify the orientation of bends, as well as making them less acute and facilitating observation inside the lumen.

At the same time, since the fluids inside lumen move in the same direction as gravity, putting the patient in this position removes the obstacle produced by fluid in the left-side intestinal tract and dilates the right-side intestinal lumen. Insertion techniques such as the "submarine technique", in which fluid is injected to maintain the lumen space and reduce the bending angle so the scope can pass through the sigmoid colon, are based on a similar theoretical rationale.

3) Effect of the weight of the scope itself

Control of the scope is also affected by the force of gravity (the weight of the scope). When advancing past the splenic flexure, the resistance and pain felt in the supine position can usually be resolved by changing the patient position to the right lateral position. One of the reasons for this may be that the acuteness of the scope's angle of entry into the splenic flexure is reduced by the weight of the scope itself. The weight of the scope can also be utilized to control excessive extension of the scope. This weight effect is also valid in other regions.

It should be pointed out that the actions produced by changing the patient's position do not operate independently, but work together to mutually reinforce each other. Although the main patient positions are the left lateral position, supine position and right lateral position, it is also possible to use the prone position in some circumstances. Take all factors into consideration in order to select the optimal patient position at a given point in the procedure.

2. Hand pressure

Hand pressure is an attempt to minimize the warping or bending of the scope with the help of external force applied from the abdominal wall.

1) When pressing the warped scope

If the scope has already been warped, the force used to push the scope forward is diverted and may not be transmitted to the distal end. The warping of the scope may also stretch the intestinal tract excessively and fracture or perforate the wall. Applying hand pressure to try and straighten the scope can help prevent excessive stretching of the intestinal tract and assist in transmission of pushing force to the scope's distal end.

2) Controlling the recovering force of intestinal tract

The straightened intestinal tract has a tendency to return to its original curved condition due to the force generated by shortening the tract, pressure from the air inside the tract, pressure from surrounding organs such as the small intestine, or the force of an adhesion. These forces for restoring the curve can be controlled by hand pressure, which is especially effective in the case of scope insertion difficulty.

3) When changing the advancing angle

Changing the scope-advancing angle also assists insertion by preventing warping.

There is no royal road to obtaining expected effects by selecting the optimum patient position change and hand pressure because the effects vary depending on the location of the scope's distal end, the direction of scope angulation, the shape of the whole scope, and the current configuration of the intestinal tract. In the sigmoid colon, in particular, accurate perception of these factors may be the key for determining the success of insertion, saving time, and performing safe insertion with less pain.

⑥ Effectiveness of patient position change and hand pressure

Yuji Inoue

1. Patient position change

Changing the patient's position is important in colonoscopy, especially when no sedation is used. Normally, I begin the examination with the patient in the left lateral position and insert the scope as if folding the sigmoid colon using the method "by shortening the colonic fold through bending".

If the scope can be inserted as far as the descending colon without excessive stretching, then it can usually be inserted all the way to the cecum with virtually no pain, even without using a sedative or analgesic. This technique is therefore critical to painless colonoscopic insertion without using a sedative or analgesic.

Although there are cases in which it is possible to insert the scope as far as the cecum with the patient in the left lateral position the whole time, in about 80% of cases I change the patient position to the supine position after entering the sigmoid colon from the rectum above the peritoneal reflection; Ra (when folding of the sigmoid colon is difficult or, specifically, most often at the anal side of the S-top). The supine position is maintained until insertion into the cecum. This position increases the flexibility of the sigmoid colon and enables deeper insertion using the method "by shortening the colonic fold through bending".

Insertion from the hepatic flexure to the ascending colon uses the paradoxical advancement technique. If there is any problem with insertion in this section, you can try changing the patient position back to the left lateral position. This pools air in the hepatic flexure, which can then be suctioned, attenuating scope angulation and enabling smooth insertion in some cases.

Although relatively rare, there are some cases in which insertion from the splenic flexure to the deep part of the transverse colon is not possible even when hand pressure is applied. In such a case, changing the patient position to the right lateral position can sometimes make the angle of the splenic flexure less acute and facilitate insertion.

In general, the three patient position changes described above are effective in most cases. However, there are occasions when random patient position changes can be effective — for example, when insertion is difficult due to adhesion. It is therefore recommended to try various patient position changes whenever you have difficulty in scope insertion.

2. Hand pressure

Hand pressure is also very important for painless colonoscopic insertion without using sedative or analgesic. What should be kept in mind here is that hand pressure should be used when the scope cannot be inserted deeper because the rectum forms a loop. There is no point in using hand pressure, however, if it causes the patient more pain than that caused by the loop formation.

The key is to find the location where hand pressure is most effective with least force, or pinpoint compression if possible. Meanwhile, the endoscopist should insert the scope using the least force to obtain the desired effect with minimum hand pressure. In my opinion, hand pressure

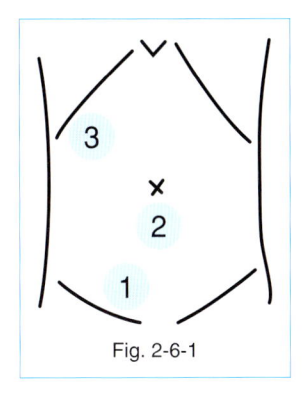

Fig. 2-6-1

is not a routine procedure but should only be applied in the following three situations: ① when folding of the sigmoid colon is difficult, ② when the sigmoid colon forms a loop that interferes with insertion into the middle of the transverse colon, and ③ when inserting the scope from the hepatic flexure to ascending colon.

1) When folding of the sigmoid colon is difficult:

When folding of the sigmoid colon becomes difficult during scope insertion into the sigmoid colon using the method "by shortening the colonic fold through bending", I first change the patient position to the supine position as described above. If shortening is still difficult, I apply hand pressure. The hand pressure location is the point where the sigmoid colon looks closest in the image, usually the superior edge of the pubis or its right side (**Fig. 2-6-1,** ①). This is the typical case in which pinpoint hand pressure is effective, and the scope should be inserted using less force than the hand pressure force. If the hand pressure does not help a different point should be compressed. A skilled endoscopist gets good at finding the most effective hand pressure point without moving the scope at all.

2) When the sigmoid colon forms a loop interfering with insertion into the middle of the transverse colon:

If the scope has Variable Stiffness capability, try increasing the stiffness. If the sigmoid colon still forms a loop, apply hand pressure in order to prevent sagging of the transverse colon (**Fig. 2-6-1,** ②).

3) When inserting the scope from the hepatic flexure to the ascending colon:

The effective hand pressure point in this case is also the point where the ascending colon looks closest in the image (**Fig. 2-6-1,** ③). If a loop is still formed, while preventing sagging of the transverse colon in the same way as 2) above, insert the scope into the ascending colon so that the scope forms a shape of letter "M", then pull back the scope slightly and let it form an upward convex shape. This will allow the scope to be inserted all the way to the cecum at once.

7 Basic hand pressure points

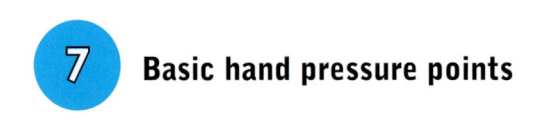

Sumio Tsuda

There are six basic hand pressure points including: (A) lower abdominal midline; (B) right lower abdomen; (C) left lower abdomen; (D) left hypochondrium; (E) upper abdominal midline; (F) right hypochondrium (**Fig. 2-7-1**). The applicability and effectiveness of each of these points is outlined below.

(A) Lower abdominal midline
This point is immediately above the pubic symphysis. Hand pressure at this point supports the shortening maneuver without stretching the sigmoid colon. In addition, it can facilitate scope manipulation when the sigmoid colon sags to the front of the rectum (indicated by the arrow in **Fig. 2-7-2**).

(B) Right lower abdomen
This point is around the center of the line connecting the anterior superior iliac spine and the umbilicus. Hand pressure is effective when the scope cannot be advanced by pushing because the sigmoid colon has formed a big loop. As the hand pressure creates a fulcrum for applying force to the scope, allowing it to be advanced, it is usually most effective to compress the anal side of the loop rather than the top.

(C) Left lower abdomen
This point corresponds to the proximity of the SD junction (SDJ). Hand pressure here attenuates the acuteness of the SDJ and facilitates entry of the scope. It also aids insertion into the intestinal tract which follows a complex contour near the SDJ (indicated by the arrow in **Fig. 2-7-3**).

(D) Left hypochondrium

This point is in the left subcostal area. Hand pressure is effective when the transverse colon follows a complex contour near the splenic flexure (indicated by the arrow in **Fig. 2-7-4**).

(E) Upper abdominal midline

This point is located above the umbilicus. Hand pressure helps prevent formation of a γ-loop in the transverse colon.

(F) Right hypochondrium

This point is in the right subcostal area. Hand pressure is effective when the transverse colon follows a complex contour near the hepatic flexure (indicated by the arrow in **Fig. 2-7-5**) or when there is an adhesion in the right side of the transverse colon due to a surgery in the upper abdomen.

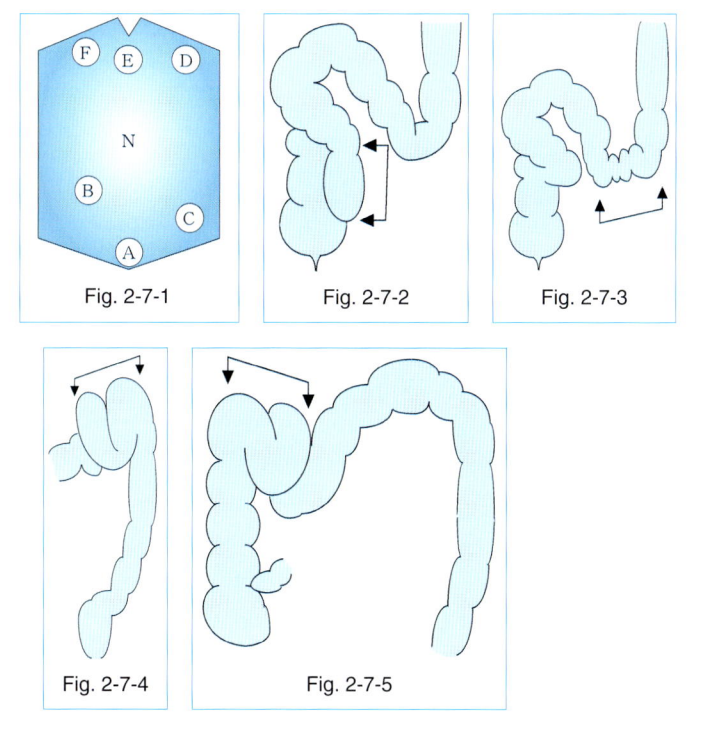

Fig. 2-7-1

Fig. 2-7-2

Fig. 2-7-3

Fig. 2-7-4

Fig. 2-7-5

3. Using a Sliding Tube

3. Using a Sliding Tube

① Advantages, disadvantages and precautions when using a sliding tube

Masahiro Igarashi

1. Advantages and disadvantages of the use of sliding tube (ST)

Advantages:
- Prevention of loop re-formation and sagging.
- Elimination of gas in the intestinal tract.
- Eases re-insertion of the scope into the right–side colon.
- Eases collection and treatment of the polyp after polypectomy.

Disadvantages:
- Contamination of examination table with drained fluid.
- Limited working length of the scope.
- Complexity of procedure means an assistant is required.
- Not necessarily indispensable.

These points should be taken into consideration when planning to use the ST.

2. How to use the ST

Fig. 3-1-1 shows how to use the ST. After removing the loop and

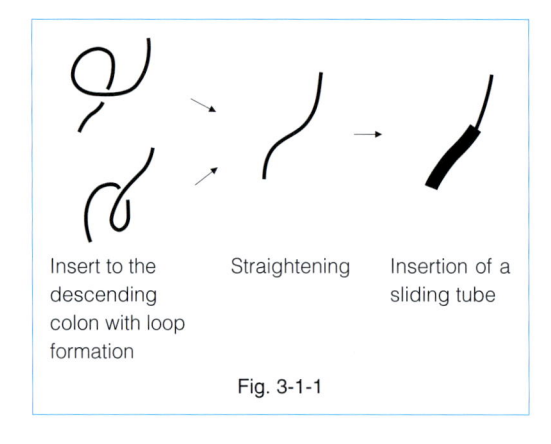

| Insert to the descending colon with loop formation | Straightening | Insertion of a sliding tube |

Fig. 3-1-1

straightening the sigmoid colon, apply lubricant jelly to the distal end and outer side of the ST and insert it gently into the oral side while rotating the distal end in both directions. When doing this, it is important to ensure that the tube is smooth by putting olive oil or the like inside it beforehand.

Be sure to hold the scope firmly so that it does not move during insertion of the ST. If the scope is pushed in while the ST is being inserted, the loop might re-form or the sigmoid colon might warp, making ST insertion more difficult. For safety, it is recommended to insert the ST under fluoroscopy so that you can have a better idea of what you are doing.

The reference position for ST insertion is at a point just past the SD junction, which corresponds to the region after the rim of the ilium in the fluoroscopic view. Note that inserting the ST too far makes it difficult to control the scope's distal end, while not inserting it far enough can result in re-formation of loop or warping of the sigmoid colon.

3. Precautions when using the ST

A typical mishap that can occur when using the ST is to leave it inserted in the patient's body. This is more likely to happen with an elderly patient with a loose anal sphincter if the endoscopist pushes in the scope too hard and the assistant does not hold the anal side of the ST firmly. If this happens, withdraw the ST by grasping it with a snare or inflating the balloon inside the ST and then pulling it out together with the scope.

② Indications for sliding tube

Yuji Inoue

1. Is a sliding tube necessary for colonoscopic insertion?

The sliding tube is used primarily when inserting a scope in the transverse colon, in cases where deep insertion is being obstructed by a loop formed by the sigmoid colon.

I seldom use a sliding tube for the following reasons: ① the sliding tube has to be put on the scope at the beginning of the procedure (there is also a detachable sliding tube but putting it on is complicated) and is uncomfortable; ② the sliding tube decreases the available effective scope length (in the dolichocolon where the sliding tube is most useful, the decreased scope length sometimes makes insertion more difficult than usual); ③ the content of the intestinal tract flows outside the patient's body after insertion of the sliding tube; and ④ the sliding tube often damages the mucosa.

However, in one or two of the 1,000 to 1,500 examinations I perform a year, I find myself forced to use a sliding tube when unable to control loop formation of the sigmoid colon using position changes and hand pressure.

The following points should be kept in mind when inserting the sliding tube: ① apply sufficient lubricant to the sliding tube to prevent damage to the intestinal tract; ② insert the sliding tube slowly while rotating it and if resistance is felt during insertion, jiggle the scope until it can be advanced without resistance; and, ③ once the tube has been inserted, have the examination technician hold it firmly so that it will not slip inside the rectum.

In the four years since Olympus developed Variable Stiffness scopes, I have never used the sliding tube in a standard colonoscopic insertion case nor experienced a case where insertion up to the cecum was difficult due to the loop formed by the sigmoid colon. In my opinion, the sliding tube is now virtually irrelevant in current colonoscopy (I usually use scopes with relatively wide diameters and Variable Stiffness capabilities such as Olympus CF-H260AZI, CF-H260AI and CF-Q240AI).

2. Indications for sliding tube in my case

At present, I only use the sliding tube for decompression of ileus cases caused by colon cancer produced on the oral side of the sigmoid colon-descending colon junction (SD junction).

Anal insertion of an ileus tube is performed as follows: ① First, insert an ordinary colonoscope proximate to the lesion, inject a contrast agent from the biopsy port of the scope and confirm the lumen. ② Next, starting at the lumen where the carcinoma is located, insert the guidewire as far as the oral side of the lesion (as close as possible to the oral side), while confirming the guidewire's movement and position with fluoroscopy. ③ Then insert the sliding tube along the scope as far as the sigmoid colon-descending colon junction (SD junction). ④ Once this is done, withdraw the scope and insert the ileus tube (although I use a system that does not require a dilator, if a dilator is required, insert the dilator before inserting the ileus tube).

A detachable sliding tube is indispensable for this operation. If an ordinary sliding tube is used, it won't be possible to remove the sliding tube after inserting the ileus tube. I once accidentally inserted an ileus tube from the anus using an ordinary sliding tube, producing erosion around the anus before the actual procedure.

③ When is the sliding tube applicable?

Hiroyuki Tsukagoshi

In general, the sliding tube is no longer used because it is not necessary. If the sliding tube is used, it may be in one of the following cases:
① When the scope is warped in spite of patient position change and hand pressure
② When deaeration of the rectum is necessary because of too much air
③ When a multiple number of large polyps are present in the deep part of the colon and need to be resected and retrieved.

1. When the scope is warped

Even when the scope is warped, insertion is still possible in most cases with the help of patient position change and hand pressure. If an assistant is not available to apply hand pressure, using a sliding tube can help make it possible to reach the cecum. The sliding tube can also be helpful for a less experienced endoscopist who uses a slim scope. However, it is not recommended as it makes it more difficult to learn the correct insertion technique.

One situation where use of a sliding tube is usually unavoidable is when the patient is obese and has an elongated sigmoid colon, as this can warp the scope and prevent it from being inserted deeply. If the abdominal wall is too thick to allow the force applied by hand pressure to be transmitted, then there is no choice but to use the sliding tube.

The thing to be careful about when using a sliding tube is that forcing it could snag some mucosa in the space between the scope and sliding tube and damage it. Considering this, if you feel any resistance, gently move the sliding tube back and forth and insert it slowly while twisting it clockwise and counterclockwise.

During insertion, check that the scope is not forming a loop. If there is no way to straighten the scope, then you will have to forego use of the sliding tube. If you are able to insert the sliding tube properly, have your assistant hold it so that it will not slip out or penetrate too deeply.

2. When deaeration is necessary

Some endoscopists attach a short sliding tube permanently to remove air. However, the real problem is the use of too much air and what such endoscopists need to do is to master the correct insertion technique as described in Chapter 1. However, if you are still a novice and have trouble decreasing the amount of air, inserting a sliding tube into the rectum will enable exhaustion of a large amount of air and facilitate scope maneuvering.

3. When retrieving polyps

There are occasions when a sliding tube is left inserted while the scope is inserted several times to retrieve a resected polyp. However, once you have become fairly skilled at scope insertion, you should have no problem inserting the scope several times without using the sliding tube. Today, with the growing availability of polyp retrieval nets, the sliding tube is rarely used for this purpose.

④ Tips on use of the sliding tube

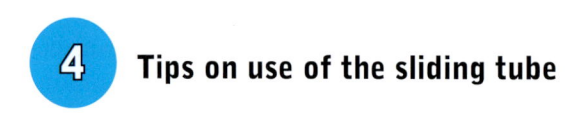

Norihiro Hamamoto

1. Insert slowly while rotating the tube

The main purpose of the sliding tube is to prevent warping of the sigmoid colon after the scope has reached the splenic flexure. Use of the sliding tube has been declining since the advent of Variable Stiffness scopes, but it can still be useful when the patient being examined has a long sigmoid colon that tends to loop easily or when hand pressure does not work. When inserting a sliding tube, let the patient know what you are doing and insert it slowly while twisting it clockwise and counterclockwise.

If the sigmoid colon is extremely long, a loop may re-form even after one has been eliminated and a tube has been inserted. In such a case, withdraw the tube, eliminate the loop, and insert the tube again. At this time, the tube must actually be inserted to an intestinal position that is deeper than before.

The sliding tube is also effective when inserting the scope again for a polypectomy after retrieving a polyp already resected by a previous polypectomy in the right side of the colon. It is not necessary, however, if retrieval by suction using a suction trap is possible.

2. Effective deaeration and warp prevention

The sliding tube effectively removes excess air as far as the descending colon, as well as preventing warping. In many cases, sufficient deaeration makes insertion into the transverse colon easy.

However, once a sliding tube has been inserted, the scope becomes much less maneuverable and there's a risk of snagging some intestinal mucosa in the tube will during the pullback operation. Therefore, it's a good idea to withdraw the tube immediately after reaching the splenic flexure.

There are some cases in which the sigmoid colon gets warped again during insertion from the hepatic flexure to the ascending colon, and the tube may have to be re-inserted in such cases. Once in a while, the entire tube has been known to enter the rectum when the endoscopist is concentrating on scope insertion while the tube is attached. Though this is quite rare, it is a good idea to attach a stopper to the tube beforehand.

3. Determine applicability based on rectal examination and abdominal palpation before insertion

It is not necessary to use the sliding tube in every case. Always perform abdominal palpation immediately before examination and attach the sliding tube only when hand pressure seems to be ineffective with the patient (such as a male with a lot of visceral fat).

On the other hand, if it is discovered during the rectal examination that the patient has a very severe anal strain or a highly developed hemorrhoid, the sliding tube should not be used.

4. Be careful not to snag the intestinal mucosa

The most important thing to avoid during the tube insertion is damage for the intestinal mucosa. Forced insertion should be avoided because it can result in intestinal perforation. Some experience is necessary to get a feel for when the degree of resistance is too great to permit further pushing. Insertion should not be forced when the resistance is high and/or when the patient complains of pain. Remember that it is not necessary to use the sliding tube in every case and that, even when a tube is attached, it does not always have to be inserted. Keep in mind that the tube is the last resort, and should only be used when hand pressure and patient position change are ineffective.

⑤ Effective use of the sliding tube

Osamu Tsuruta, Hiroshi Kawano

Of the approximately 2500 total colonoscopic examinations are conducted at our facility each year using the one-man technique with medium-length colonoscopes and without fluoroscopy (nor UPD), there are one or two in which the cecum cannot be reached without fluoroscopy and a full examination is not possible unless a sliding tube is used under fluoroscopy.

There are also cases in which the sliding tube can be used to retrieve a large polyp after polypectomy. We will describe how to use the sliding tube in both cases.

1. Effective use of sliding tube during insertion (Fig. 3-5-1)

When the descending colon is not fixed on the posterior peritoneum, it is sometimes not possible to advance the distal end of the inserted scope toward the oral side once the scope reaches a point just past the Rs-S junction, and only the sigmoid colon is pushed up toward the cranial side

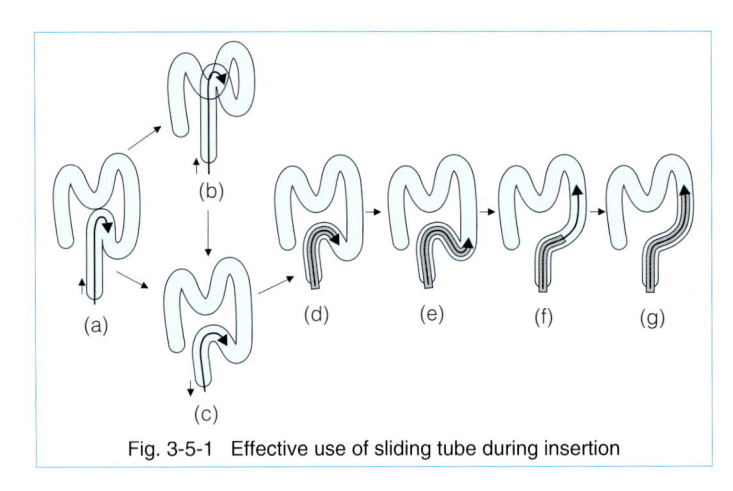

Fig. 3-5-1 Effective use of sliding tube during insertion

(b).

If this happens, pull the scope out under fluoroscopy and make the Rs-S junction as flat as possible (c), and insert the siding tube as far as the anal side of the sigmoid colon (d). The scope can then be inserted and advanced toward the oral side because the S-top is kept in place by the sliding tube (e).

After advancing beyond the SD junction, pull the scope to straighten it and advance it into the descending colon (f). From there, advance the distal end a little at a time by pushing and pulling the scope. As the scope advances, insert the sliding tube together with it until it reaches the proximity of the splenic flexure (g). Now, secure the sliding tube in that position and manipulate the scope, which can be advanced easily toward the oral side.

2. Retrieval of large polyp (Fig. 3-5-2)

A large endoscopically resected lesion/polyp can be hard to retrieve because it cannot pass through the anal canal. This is not a problem if a retrieval net is available; if not, the sliding tube can be used.

First move the resected polyp to the rectum, then remove the scope temporarily, attach a sliding tube to the scope and insert the scope and sliding tube into the rectum. After insertion, grasp the polyp using a 5-prong forceps (or similar instrument) under endoscopic observation, pull part (a) or all (b) of the polyp into the sliding tube, then withdraw the scope and sliding tube together through the anal canal.

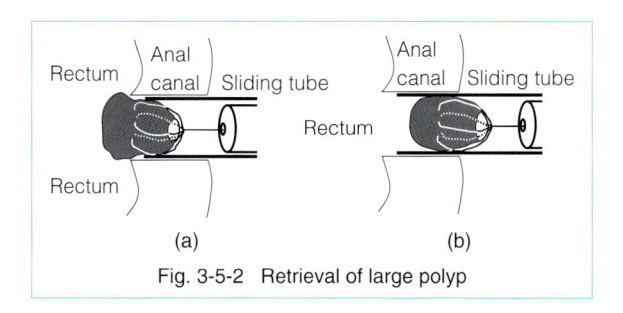

Fig. 3-5-2 Retrieval of large polyp

4. Insertion into the Rectum

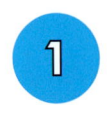

① Select a scope appropriate to the patient

Takahisa Matsuda

In upper gastrointestinal endoscopy, it is rarely necessary to have to choose what type of scope to use. In colonoscopy, on the other hand, various types of scope are available — including the thin scope, Variable Stiffness scope and magnifying scope — and it is important to select the one that is most appropriate to the purpose of the examination and the specifics of the patient.

The thin scope is suitable for patients who have had a laparotomy and appear to have adhesions as well as for insertion through a stoma, while the combination of a Variable Stiffness scope and UPD may work best with patients with dolichocolon.

1. Carefully insert the scope from the anus into the rectum

After performing a rectal examination to observe the anus and proximate regions, insert the scope slowly from the anus into the rectum.

There are two reasons why the insertion should be slow and careful. One is the possibility of anal pain caused by a hemorrhoid or other problem. It is important to avoid causing the patient any pain at this point as this could make them wary of deep insertion. The other reason is the possibility that a lesion may be present on the anterior wall of the lower rectum (Rb), which may bleed when it is contacted by the scope. If a lesion is present that requires detailed invasion diagnosis with magnifying observation, special care is required because bleeding makes accurate observation impossible.

2. Scope insertion technique

It is commonly believed that the most difficult part of colonoscope insertion is the SD junction. However, when using the technique "by shortening the colonic fold through bending," it should be emphasized that the complexities of insertion begin at the rectum.

The examination starts with the patient in the left lateral position. After insertion into the rectum (Rb), suction enough air to ease scope passage and advance it using counterclockwise rotation. The scope should not be advanced exclusively by pushing, but should be inserted with the idea of squeezing each and every fold in the intestinal tract. Be careful not to insufflate in too much air, but also be careful not to absorb any mucosa when suctioning as this could cause peristalsis of the intestinal tract.

As the scope is advanced for the most part using counterclockwise rotation, it will usually be necessary to switch the scope toward the right at about 20 cm from the AV. Around the time your hand starts to feel free after switching to the right, a sharp bend toward the right will be felt. This point is the S-top position.

We call this position the S-top because we believe that this position corresponds to the highest point of the sigmoid colon in the N-loop. In most cases, the patient position is changed from the left lateral position to the supine position once the scope has been inserted to this point. The key is to pass the S-top by shortening it without stretching.

② Help the patient relax and get the information you need to perform insertion

Norihiro Hamamoto

1. What should be done before performing an examination?

Before beginning your examination, make sure you talk with the patient first in order to make them feel more comfortable and to obtain the information you need to perform a successful insertion. Greet the patient, confirm their name, check their experience of abdominal surgery, and ask them to let you know immediately if they experience any pain.

While you are doing this, observe the patient's physique and physical condition. Also, perform a palpation of the abdomen to identify whether sliding tube insertion might be necessary and what scope that would be most effective for the patient. With a male patient who has excessive visceral fat that may make hand pressure ineffective, it is recommended to attach a sliding tube onto the scope. A slim scope is suitable for thin women and older patients.

Put the patient in the left lateral position and tell them that you are starting the rectal examination. Do not insert your finger abruptly as this is enough to make the patient overly tense. Apply sufficient lubricant to the anus and palpate the region from the anal canal to the lower rectum. Then insert the scope slowly. Sometimes I use my left elbow to compress the suprapubic or right hypochondrium region. In this case, I put the monitor in front of me and position myself parallel to the bed. Hand pressure can be applied by an assistant if it is difficult to do it yourself, although it's often easier to accurately manipulate the scope when hand pressure is performed by the endoscopist rather than by an assistant.

To improve your sensitivity to the resistance transmitted by the scope, gently grasp the shaft with the thumb and index finger of the right hand, while resting you other fingers where comfortable without applying any pressure. During examination, always be aware of the scope axis and always try to hold a section at 20 to 40 cm from the anus in order to maintain high torque tracking.

2. Manipulate the scope as if swinging it to the left and right, rather than pushing

The approach from the rectum insertion to the S-top position is critical in determining how smoothly subsequent insertion will proceed. If air is insufflated carelessly during this stage, the subsequent procedure will be extremely difficult. If the scope were advanced through a bend by exclusively pushing it while insufflating air, a loop would likely form in the extent after the S-top. The trick is to reach the S-top linearly by the shortest distance using as little air as possible. Use meticulous care for insertion even if it takes longer.

The key to successful insertion is make good use of the "slalom" technique. Ideally, you would pass the scope through the intestinal tract by twisting the scope clockwise and counterclockwise while gently applying upward angulation to the intestinal folds and moving the scope axis to the left and right. Do not push the scope; instead, manipulate the scope as if swinging it to the left and right while maintaining a minimum distance so that the distal end does not contact the intestinal wall.

Although the scope is actually advancing, you will not feel a pushing sensation because you are actually twisting the scope clockwise and counterclockwise. Until you reach the S-top, you will mainly be twisting in the counterclockwise direction. When you encounter an acute bend at the 3 o'clock direction, it means the scope has reached the position between rectosigmoid (RS) and S-top. Now, change the patient to the supine position and start the approach from the S-top to the SD junction.

③ Things that should be done before insertion

Hiroshi Kashida

1. Patient posture and arrangement of the light source and monitor

Usually, the patient should be placed in the left lateral position with the hip and knee joints bent almost at right angles before starting examination.

If it is not possible to put the patient in this position because of a curved spine, bone fracture or hemiplegia, have the patient select a more comfortable position. If the patient has an artificial anus, it is best to start the examination in the supine position. If the height of the examination table can be adjusted, adjust it according to the height of the endoscopist.

The layout of the light source and monitor can differ at different institutes; **Fig. 4-3-1** shows the layout used at our department.

2. Digital anal examination is also important

Apply Xylocaine Jelly® to an index finger and perform a digital anal examination. The purposes of this examination are described below:

① Since most rectal cancers are located within the reach of a finger, inserting a scope blindly could damage the lesion or cause bleeding, making it necessary to get some idea in advance. The digital examination also makes it possible to identify the tightness of the anus and the presence of hemorrhoids. After withdrawing the finger, check it for blood.

② Xylocaine Jelly® works as a local anesthesia for the anus and also lubricates the way so that the scope can be inserted smoothly.

③ Even when surface anesthesia is applied, the patient will reflexively try to close the anus if the scope is inserted abruptly, producing resistance to the scope or inflicting pain on the patient. When performing the digital anal examination, tell the patient before inserting your finger.

Insert the finger slowly and leave it inserted for 5 to 10 seconds; this will relax the muscle tension in the anal region. During digital examination, also check the contours of the anal canal and rectum.

Xylocaine Jelly® dries as time passes. Therefore, once the examination has started, another kind of lubricant jelly may be used. However, take care not to use too much jelly since it makes the hand slippery and scope operation difficult. As the lubricant jelly does not have an anesthetic action, Xylocaine Jelly® is preferable for the digital anal examination.

3. Do not insert the scope yet

If the scope is twisted, it can be difficult to insert. As endoscopists become more technically adept, they often check functions such as insufflation, irrigation and suction unconsciously before starting insertion, as any professionals would do before their work. Since insufflation tends to be excessive, it is recommended to set the insufflation setting at a minimum or medium position before insertion.

4. Now, begin insertion

Angulate the scope slightly upward and, while holding it with the right index finger, and slip the distal end gently into the anus, starting from the edge of the distal end. This will help minimize the pain at the anus. Once the scope has entered the rectum, the endoscopist should straighten the scope and assume an appropriate posture of him/herself before further insertion.

While suctioning residual fluids in the rectum, advance the scope, being careful to keep insufflation to a minimum. The Rs-S junction can be reached quickly because the distance is only about 10 cm if no air is insufflated.

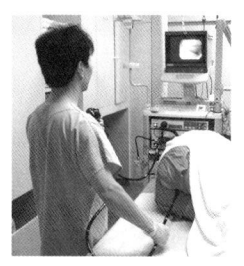

Fig. 4-3-1

④ Start with a rectal examination

Yuji Inoue

1. The importance of performing a rectal examination

Place the patient in the left lateral position, apply Xylocaine Jelly® to the index finger of your right hand and proceed with the rectal examination. Despite the name, this "rectal examination" is not a full examination. You should limit it to checking the anal canal lumen and applying jelly to that region. Performing a detailed examination up to the rectum could damage the mucosa and make it more difficult to find small lesions in the rectum. In cases where a true rectal examination is required — to check for rectal lesions or hemorrhoids, for example — it is better to do it after the colonoscopic examination. A minimal rectal examination as described above must be performed, however, because insertion into the rectum could otherwise be difficult, potentially damaging the anal mucosa and inflicting pain on the patient.

In addition, with patients who have had hemorrhoid surgery and may suffer from a narrowed anus, a preliminary rectal examination is necessary for pre-procedural checking of the lumen. If a severe stricture is found during the examination, switch to a slimmer scope if necessary. Since this "rectal examination" is the first stage of the colonoscopic examination, it is important to make the patient feel comfortable and at ease before beginning.

2. Inserting the scope into the rectum

After applying sufficient jelly inside the anal canal, lubricant should also be applied to the scope. I use jelly made for ultrasonography as a lubricant. After lubricating the scope and the anal canal, place the index finger of the right hand on the scope, gently place the scope in the proximity of the anus, insufflate air gently and insert the scope while checking the lumen. Once inside the anal canal, the scope should be inserted slightly toward the anterior side of the patient.

With a female patient, be careful not to insert the scope into the vagina. I was once referred to a 30-year female who had been diagnosed with rectal cancer with circumferential stricture by another physician. Because a friend of this woman was an acquaintance of mine, she visited me before the results of biopsy were made clear. As she was only 30 years old and had not noticed any symptoms herself, I immediately performed a colonoscopy, but could not find a tumor even by inserting the scope up to the cecum. Rectal observation was detailed and comprehensive, and repeated about 10 times, but no tumor was discovered. While I was making a reservation for a contrast-enema examination to double-check my results, I received a report from the physician who had referred her to me, saying that the results of the biopsy showed that the specimen was part of the uterine epithelium. I asked the patient for confirmation, but she said that she was so tense during the examination that she did not notice the incorrect insertion at all.

In fact, while monitoring colonoscopies from monitoring rooms, I have occasionally observed trainees mistakenly inserting the scope into the vagina. However, the differentiation should be very easy (and possible right at the moment of insertion) because the color tone inside the normal rectum is reddish while that inside the vagina is whitish.

As already mentioned, the scope should be inserted toward the anterior side of the patient from the anal canal. These mistakes may be the result of focusing too much on frontward insertion, as well as applying too much jelly.

3. Rotating the scope inside rectum

After entering the rectum, advance the scope by rotating it counterclockwise, and then enter the upper rectum by rotating it clockwise. It is important to insert the scope as if pulling the lumen toward you while securing the lumen by keeping insufflation to a minimum.

A skilled endoscopist can identify a difficult case immediately after insertion into the rectum. It has been my experience that when the rectum looks as if it has been folded, it frequently poses insertion difficulties because of dolichocolon.

⑤ "Catching the bend"

Satoru Tamura

Before inserting the scope, anesthetize the anal canal surface with Xylocaine Jelly® to make it slippery and enable smooth insertion into the rectum. Be careful not to insert your finger as deeply as you would in a rectal examination as this causes reddening on the rectal mucosa and makes it difficult to differentiate it from a lesion.

When the scope is inserted with the patient in the left lateral position, the scope will hit the anterior wall and the image turns completely red. Since the rectum runs along the flexure on the front of the sacrum, withdraw the scope slightly, angulate it upward and insert it into the ampulla of the rectum below the peritoneal reflection (Rb) by rotating it slightly counterclockwise.

Three transverse folds of the rectum (Houston's valves) can be observed when the scope enters Rb. The inferior and middle rectal valves can be passed easily by slightly rotating the scope clockwise and counterclockwise to reach the superior rectal valve. The superior rectal valve usually constitutes a leftward bend and enters the rectosigmoid; Rs (Rs as recognized by endoscopy), which can be passed by angulating the scope upward to catch the bending section with the distal end (**Fig. 4-5-1**), and then rotating the scope counterclockwise while pulling it a little. If this section is passed using the push move exclusively, a bend will form a loop so it is very important to start the shortening move from this initial bend. Nevertheless, there are some cases in which this bend forms an extremely acute angle, thereby making it hard to catch the folds.

If the scope cannot be advanced and time is being wasted, it is important to have a skilled endoscopist take over the procedure. Whether or not this section can be passed by shortening will determine how easily the scope can be subsequently advanced in the sigmoid colon.

If shortening is impossible in spite of every effort made, an alternative method is to identify the contour of the intestinal tract, confirm the absence of resistance and push to advance the scope's distal end slightly until the next lumen ("slide-by-mucosa" technique). However, if the monitor image turns white during this operation, it means there is a risk of perforation. This technique is not recommended for patients with diverticulosis, inflammatory bowel disease or severe adhesion. Novices should focus their attention on mastering the basic techniques and refrain from attempting to use an alternative technique whenever possible.

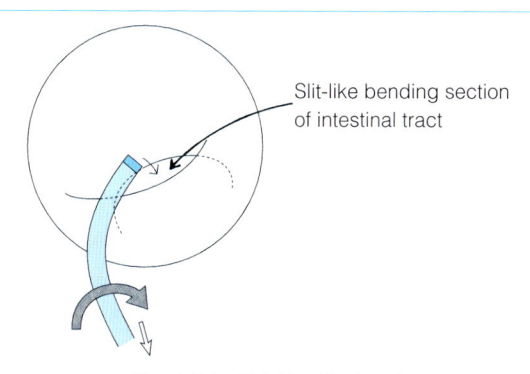

Fig. 4-5-1   Catching the bend

This is the first step of the shortening move for insertion of colonoscope. The clearance available in the bending section of intestinal tract is not always sufficient, often being no more than a narrow slit.

The technique I use here is what I call "catching the bend", which involve sliding the scope's distal end into the slit and hooking the bend. To do this, first suction out enough air to soften the angle of the bend. Then, with the scope angulated slightly upward, bring the distal end close to the bend.

The important thing here is the distance between the scope and the intestinal wall in front of it. If there is not enough space, the scope image turns completely red. If there is too much space, catching the bend will be impossible. Maintain an optimum distance, while sliding the scope in by rotating it. Once this procedure is accomplished, you can proceed to the next step, for example, pulling the next bend toward you or passing a bend by rotating the scope.

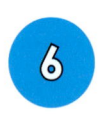

Insertion into the anus, passage through the anal canal and rectum, and observation of these regions

Osamu Tsuruta, Hiroshi Kawano

1. Patient position

We put the patient in the left lateral position for insertion. The reason is that this position best facilitates naked-eye observation of the anal region before insertion, digital rectal examination and scope insertion into the anal canal.

2. Naked-eye observation of the anus and proximity

Before insertion, check for the presence of perianal skin lesions, anal fistula, hemorrhoids, etc., with the naked eye.

3. Digital rectal examination

Before insertion, perform a digital rectal examination to check for the presence of anal stenosis, anal canal lesions and lower rectal (Rb) lesions.

If the anal canal is narrow, select a slim scope. If a lesion appears to be present in the anal canal, observe the anal canal carefully during scope insertion. If a tumor growth is detected in Rb, insert the scope more slowly and cautiously than usual to prevent bleeding due to contact with the scope.

A digital rectal examination using 2% Xylocaine Jelly® also helps reduce anal pain during scope insertion and makes it easier to pass the scope through the anal canal, as well as facilitating scope manipulation such insertion, withdrawal and rotation.

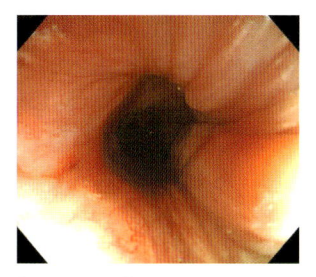

Fig. 4-6-1 Observation of the anal canal

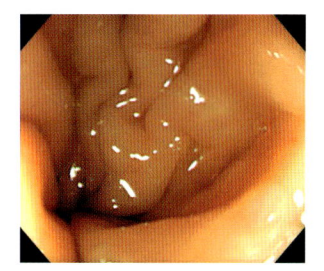

Fig. 4-6-2 Advancing the scope while avoiding the use of insufflation as much as possible

4. Scope insertion

1) Inserting into the anus

Hold the scope's distal end with the right hand, place the index finger on the scope and insert it into the anus.

2) Passing through the anal canal (**Fig. 4-6-1**)

When the scope's distal end enters the anus, insufflate air and, while observing the anal canal, advance the scope slowly. Observation during passage through the anal canal can be made easier by slightly increasing insufflation.

3) Passing through the rectum (**Fig. 4-6-2**)

Insufflation should be kept to a minimum for passage through the rectum. Excessive insufflation can stretch and dilate the rectum and sigmoid colon, making it more difficult to pass the scope through the Rs-S junction, sigmoid colon and SD junction.

When we perform a procedure, we set the air button to the low position immediately after entering the rectum from the anal canal and advance the scope, while avoiding the use of insufflation as much as possible. If some insufflation is necessary, we always try to suction it whenever possible.

As the extent from the anal canal to Rb is oriented toward the posterior side of the patient, we advance the scope by rotating the scope counterclockwise, while the patient is in the left lateral position. From there, we advance the scope to the Rs-S junction while checking the subsequent lumen by angulating the scope. To advance the scope, we rely primarily on rotation and angulation, avoiding the push move as much as possible. If pushing becomes necessary, we always add the pull-back move in order to keep the scope as straight as possible. We believe that these moves will soften the angle of the Rs-S junction and facilitate the insertion from there to the oral side.

5. Passing the Rs-S Junction

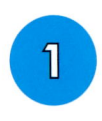

1 Passing the rectosigmoid junction using knowledge of the location's contours based on three-dimensional anatomy

Shinji Tanaka

1. Put the patient in the left lateral position to perform insertion and for observation of the rectum

Use the left lateral position for insertion into, and observation of, the rectum, as this position allows air to accumulate in the rectum. When actually inserting the scope, the trick to passing through the rectosigmoid junction lies in moving the scope to the rectosigmoid junction by insufflating the minimum amount of air in the section from Rb (the lower rectum) to Ra (above the lower rectum) and taking the shortest distance.

If too much air is insufflated or the scope is inserted in an unnatural direction between Rb and Ra, it will become more difficult to insert the scope due to excessive stretching of the rectum and sigmoid colon.

2. The importance of understanding the shape of the colon based on three-dimensional anatomy

Having an understanding of the stereo image of the colons based on three-dimensional anatomy is essential. The rectum initially runs toward the back in the section from the anus to the sacrum, then turns toward the abdomen at the Rb-Ra boundary and, though there are some variations, usually goes leftward toward the SD (sigmoid-descending) junction. The endoscopist views this three-dimensional structure from the back of the patient in the left lateral position.

Once you know the general outline of the colon, it will be obvious that the most effective means of insertion is to pass the Rb-Ra boundary and enter the rectosigmoid junction by initially rotating the scope counterclockwise. Mapping out this insertion route in your head makes it possible to estimate the direction for advancing the scope with minimum insufflation by referring to folds, even when the view is not clear.

3. Using suction rather than unnecessary insufflation

It is not unusual to encounter a fairly acute bend in the extent from Ra to Rs and the sigmoid colon. However, even in this case, if you have a good understanding of the three-dimensional anatomy of the large intestine, you will be able to insert the scope's distal end between folds and enter the sigmoid colon as if by folding the bend by rotating the scope clockwise.

At this time, it is recommended to rely on suction, rather than insufflation. This makes it possible to reach the sigmoid colon with minimum stretching of the intestinal tract (by the shortest distance).

4. The importance of being able to feel any resistance to the scope

During insertion, the optimum position for holding the scope with the right hand is always about 30 to 40 cm from the anus, though this varies depending on the stiffness of the scope. Holding the scope at distance from the anus allows the right hand to feel any slight resistance to the scope inside the patient and also helps prevent forced pushing of the scope. It is strongly recommended that colonoscopy novices hold the scope this way.

② Hooking-the-fold technique and rotation factor

Toru Mitsushima

During scope insertion, the junction between the rectum and rectosigmoid colon (Rs) in the pelvic cavity, which is fixed and immobile, and the sigmoid colon junction (Rs-S junction), which is located in the abdominal cavity and fully mobile by means of the sigmoid mesocolon, often forms a twist or acute bend and hinders smooth advancement of the scope.

In the Rs that is fully secured by the surrounding connective tissues, the intestinal tract does not rotate spontaneously and the spatial relationships between left/right and anterior/posterior walls do not change unless the scope is rotated. However, when the scope advances into the sigmoid colon, the lumen rotates freely and the positional relationship between the scope and the proximal-side intestinal wall and bend changes all the time. As a result, in the Rs-S junction, scope maneuvering needs to be flexible and quick in order to trace the rapid orientation changes of the proximal-side lumen.

When not stretched excessively by the scope or by gas, the accumulation of bends at the Rs-S junction looks like the pleats in an accordion. To advance the scope smoothly in this region, always use the following technique.

When the scope's distal end has advanced past Rs, angulate the scope upward, twist it slightly counterclockwise, and push to pass the bend toward the proximal-side lumen that develops in the 9 o'clock direction on the monitor screen. After passing the bend, keep the scope angulated upward and pull it slightly by rotating it clockwise rotation to untwist the scope and intestinal tract. Then, while keeping the scope angled upwards and rotating it slightly clockwise, push it forward. After passing the next bend, pull the scope by rotating counterclockwise, angulate it rightward and advance it by making use of its repulsion force.

This series of maneuvers is basically the same as the hooking-the-fold technique* proposed by Dr. Shinya, the difference being the element of rotation not mentioned by Dr. Shinya. In fact, I believe that in order to advance the scope smoothly, the rotation factor is essential, namely by push-advancing the scope with a counterclockwise rotation, then pulling it back with a clockwise rotation, advancing it with a clockwise rotation, pulling it back with a counterclockwise rotation and angulating it rightward (**Fig. 5-2-1**).

By repeating the above cycle a few times, the scope's distal end can be advanced past the Rs-S junction into the sigmoid colon. In patients with a short sigmoid colon, you may find that you can advance the scope to the descending colon without even being aware of the SD bends.

※ Shinya, H.: Colonoscopy, Diagnosis and Treatment of Colonic Disease. Igakushoin, Tokyo, 1982

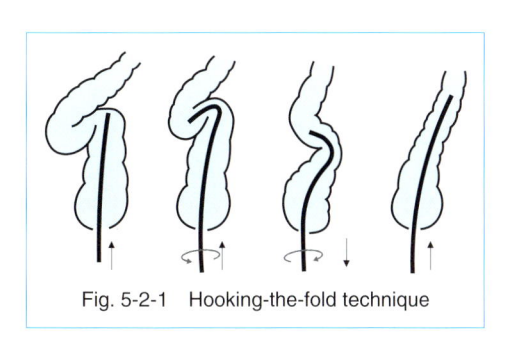

Fig. 5-2-1　Hooking-the-fold technique

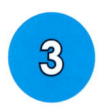

③ Effective use of patient position changes and external abdominal compression

Takahisa Matsuda

1. Basic method for passing the S–top

The crucial stage in colonoscope insertion is the RS-S junction (at the position in the bend close to the S-top at around 20 cm AV). If the intestinal tract is stretched here, a loop could form or the scope could warp, causing the patient pain. In cases where shortening is easy, the left lateral position can be maintained during folding, but in most cases I change the patient position to the supine position because shortening is usually easier in this position.

The shortening operation can be facilitated by applying external abdominal compression, as well as by changing the patient position. The assistant can determine the compression site by observing the video monitor to locate the point where the bend is closest to the scope. Typically, this point is in the lower abdominal or suprapupic area. Theoretically, compression should be applied from the upward direction so that the S-top does not stretch upward (**Fig. 5-3-1**).

As compression is being applied, the endoscopist moves the scope to the bend by slightly angulating the distal end upward, while keeping the scope ready to pull. To pass the S-top, imagine that you are sliding the scope into the bend with downward angulation, while applying rightward rotation force. The important thing here is to apply the angulation and rotation forces slowly, just a little at a time.

If the intestinal tract cannot be shortened even with external abdominal compression (which may occur in a case involving adhesion due to laparotomy or in a case with a high S-top), you can try putting the patient in the right lateral position and performing the technique described above. Keep in mind that pushing to shorten the tract after a loop is formed should always be the last resort. If the S-top can be passed by shortening without stretching, the scope can be advanced straight without being affected by any bend in the SD junction created when an N-shaped loop is formed.

2. Evaluating patient pain

At our facility, both insertion time and the degree of patient discomfort are noted on the endoscopic examination result sheet. Patient discomfort is categorized in three levels: (A) insertion without any pain; (B) pain that the patient can manage; (C) analgesic or sedative required. According to the results of about 4,000 procedures performed by four endoscopists with extensive experience in colonoscopies, most patients experienced little or no pain — 71.0% (A), 22.8%(B) and 6.2% (C).

In other words, once the insertion technique "by shortening the colonic fold through bending" has been mastered, an analgesic or sedative will not be required with about 90% of patients. As the percentage of patients in group A (insertion without any pain) was about 70%, it is likely that the percentage of cases in which the right amount of shortening is achieved at the RS-S junction (S-top) may also be about 70%. Therefore, mastering the countermeasures we have described would lead to improvement of the colonoscope insertion in the remaining 30%.

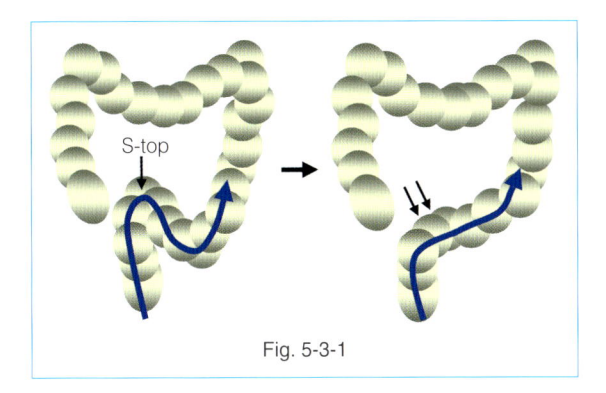

Fig. 5-3-1

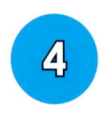

④ Getting past the Rs-S junction is the key to a successful colonoscopy

Hiroyuki Tsukagoshi

As you get used to performing colonoscopies, you will get to the point where passing the Rs-S junction is so easy, it's something you do almost unconsciously. However, despite your growing confidence, you never force anything if radiation enteritis or a severe inflammation is present. Knowing when to stop is important if you are going to avoid perforating the intestine.

Unfortunately, I have found that many people use the wrong insertion method. This applies not only to beginners, but also to experienced endoscopists. It is no exaggeration to say that the success of colonoscopy depends on using the correct method to pass the Rs-S junction. The problem is that people advance the colonoscope in the same way as an upper GI scope, that is, by insufflating air to maintain the view. This is a bad habit that is particularly common with endoscopists who have performed numerous upper GI endoscopies.

In colonoscopy, the correct way to insert the scope is to advance the colonoscope slowly, as if plowing through the mucosae, while using as little air as possible as described in Chapter 1 (page 6). The view of the lumen should never be like a drainage tile. If this can be done, it is no longer necessary to follow the traditional insertion technique, which is to rotate the scope counterclockwise to view the bend in the 12 o'clock direction, and then angulate the scope upward, and so on. The insertion technique with minimum air amount can be used in any region, allowing the endoscopist to move the scope forward without even being aware of what region the scope is passing through.

1. How to hold the scope

Endoscopists who insufflate excessive air often hold the scope with their left index finger on the suction button and their middle finger on the air button. As a result, they tend to insufflate air without even being aware of it, increasing the amount of air in the intestine. When holding a scope, make sure you do not place your finger on the air button. Instead, place the index finger on the suction button and use the other fingers to hold the scope firmly.

2. Maneuvering with minimal air

When you use only a small amount of air, it means you are going to come into close quarters with the colon. The scope is forced to move slowly, and spends more time stationary than moving. However, if, as a result of poor preparation, the colon contains a large amount of opaque fluid or solid stool, an increase in the amount of air is unavoidable. But the basic insertion method is still the same: Approach the farthest wall of a curve, bring the curve to the 12 o'clock position in the field of view, carefully align the scope orientation with the curve, and bring the next lumen into view while pulling the scope. This operation resembles that for insertion into the ileocecal valve.

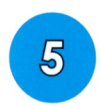

⑤ Passing through the Rs-S junction the right way is the key to success

Hiroshi Kashida

1. The trick is to pull back the scope just before the junction

The Rs-S junction usually appears on the left of the monitor image. The bend is quite sharp, so the lumen beyond is invisible. At this point, angulate the scope upward and pull it slightly, while twisting it counterclockwise as if trying to pull the rectum toward you. This will make the angle of the Rs-S junction less acute, making the sigmoid colon lumen visible on the right of the monitor. Now, straighten the scope and immediately twist it clockwise. The scope will enter the sigmoid colon as if it were drawn by gravitation (**Fig. 5-5-1**).

2. Imagine pulling an oar

When twisting the scope counterclockwise and then clockwise as described above, part of the scope is in contact with the bed. This contact point can be used as a kind of "fulcrum" to facilitate scope maneuvering (**Fig. 5-5-2**). This can be compared to rowing a traditional-style single-oared Japanese boat or an Italian gondola.

3. Do not push your way through the Rs-S junction

Sometimes, you may find it possible to push the scope through the Rs-S junction. Don't push it too much. If you push the scope and the Rs-S junction is stretched, the sigmoid colon is likely to form a large loop toward the right or cranial side, thereby making subsequent passage of the SD junction difficult. While all endoscopists are very careful when passing the SD junction, it might be too late because success here depends on how the Rs-S junction was passed before it.

Fig. 5-5-1

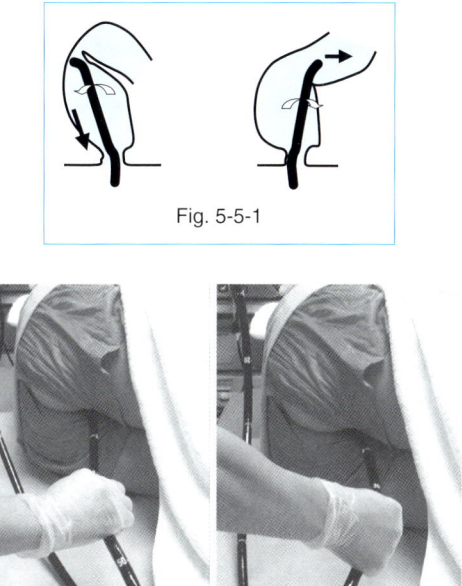

Fig. 5-5-2

6 Tips on passage through the Rs-S junction

Yusuke Saitoh

Important points to remember
- Since the subsequent lumen is most often visible in the 6 to 8 o'clock direction, this region should be navigated using the hooking-the-fold technique by twisting the scope counterclockwise.
- Never attempt to push the scope through the Rs-S junction.
- Suction excess air from the rectum.

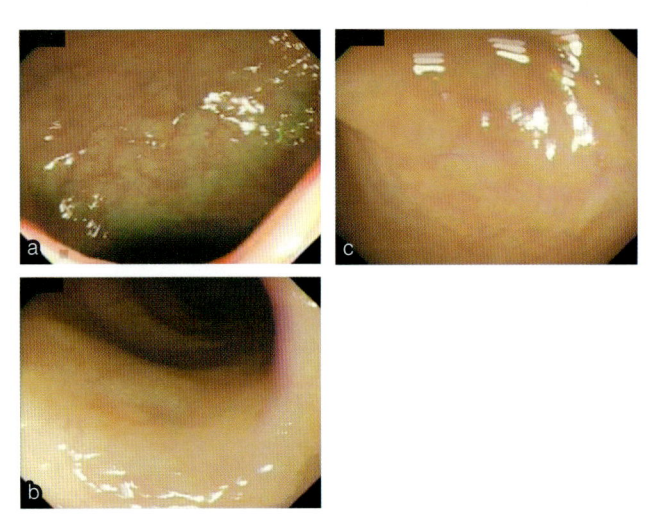

Fig. 5-6-1　Passage through Rs-S junction
a) The lumen of the Rs-S junction is usually visible in the 6 to 8 o'clock direction.
b) Twist the scope counterclockwise so that the lumen can be viewed in the 12 o'clock direction (the photo shows the view in the middle of counterclockwise rotation so the subsequent lumen is visible in the 9 o'clock direction).
c) When the scope is advanced using the hooking-the-fold technique with upward angulation, the sigmoid colon lumen is visible on the right.

Along with the SD junction, the Rs-S junction is one of the most critical points in scope insertion. When the scope reaches this region, the subsequent lumen is usually visible in the 6 to 8 o'clock direction (**Fig. 5-6-1a**). To pass the junction, twist the scope counterclockwise and adjust it so that the fold of the Rs-S junction is visible in the 12 o'clock direction (**Fig. 5-6-1b**).

Enter the sigmoid colon angulating the scope upwards, while using the hooking-the-fold technique (one of the most important techniques of the one-man method, in which the scope is advanced by hooking a mucosal fold with the scope's distal end and then pulling the scope, reducing the angle of the bend to smooth the scope's passage).

The lumen of the sigmoid colon usually comes into view on the right (**Fig. 5-6-1c**). **Never try to push the scope through this region** as it perforates easily, and if it is stretched too much, it can easily form a double loop when the scope reaches the SD junction. It is also helpful to suction any excess air in the rectum before passing through the Rs-S junction, as this will make it easier to pass through the sigmoid colon and SD junction.

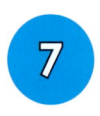

7 The trick is to reduce the amount of air in the rectum

Hiro-o Yamano

Let us take a look at the first bend we encounter after the scope is inserted through the anus. If there is too much air in the rectum, it can make the subsequent procedure more difficult by preventing you from shortening the sigmoid colon enough to move the scope forward. Suction of the residual intestinal fluids is of course necessary, but the key point is to eliminate as much air in the rectum as possible.

In general, the sigmoid colon can be entered by angulating the scope slightly upward from Ra (rectum above the peritoneal reflection), while rotating it counterclockwise so that its distal end points toward the left side of the patient. Once the scope is inside the sigmoid colon, you can shorten the colon using the clockwise torque of the scope.

In rare cases, the lumen after Ra may be reachable with clockwise torque from Ra, that is, toward the right side of the patient. In this case, the scope should be advanced into the sigmoid colon following the contours of the lumen, that is, by rotating the scope clockwise for a short period. Be sure not to do this for too long as this insertion method will eventually cause a loop formation. It is important to switch the rotation direction counterclockwise at the earliest possible opportunity.

6. Passing the SD Junction

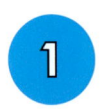

① The two basic SD junction passage techniques that need to be mastered

Sumio Tsuda

The SD junction (SDJ) is the most difficult section to get past when inserting a colonoscope. A variety of techniques have been developed that promise to get the endoscopist past this point, two of which should be mastered by all endoscopists: 1) passing the SDJ while shortening it from the sigmoid colon; 2) passing the SDJ by pushing the scope from the sigmoid colon.

1. Passing the SDJ while shortening it from the sigmoid colon

This technique involves rotating the scope both clockwise and counterclockwise to advance it through the sigmoid colon without pushing, which could result in excessive stretching of the sigmoid colon. Finally, rotate the scope clockwise to reach the SDJ. To pass the SDJ, the endoscopist also rotates the scope. In other words, this technique works by shortening the intestinal tract exclusively via scope rotations, while keeping the scope straight whenever possible.

To make this technique easier, change the patient position from the left lateral position to the supine position when the scope's distal end has passed the rectosigmoid junction and then apply pressure to the point immediately above the pubic symphysis. The key to the success of this method is to avoid excessive insufflation and manipulate the scope slowly.

2. Passing the SDJ by pushing the scope from the sigmoid colon

Although passing the SDJ by shortening it from the sigmoid colon as described above is normally the best option, it is not applicable in all cases. If shortening is not possible, then the endoscopist will have to push the scope through the SDJ. In this case, insert the scope's distal end into the region between the descending colon and splenic flexure by forming an N-loop or α-loop.

Because the push operation presents a high risk of causing the patient to suffer pain and discomfort, it is important to be very careful and take precautions. Avoid excessive stretching of the intestinal tract with unnecessary insufflation, use hand pressure to help advance the scope, switch to the pull-back operation when necessary to decrease loop size, always move the scope slowly, and so on. Administration of a sedative should also be considered as required.

After the scope has been inserted by pushing, the scope must be straightened. This is done by rotating and pulling the scope shaft, but it is important to keep the scope's distal end at a point beyond the SDJ while you are doing this. From a safety point of view, a slim scope is suitable for push-type insertion.

② Take the configuration of the sigmoid colon into consideration

Satoru Tamura

While there are many variations in the configuration of the sigmoid colon, they can be roughly categorized into three major patterns (**Fig. 6-2-1**). In general, regardless of the pattern, when inserting a scope, the idea is to shorten the sigmoid colon so that the SD junction can be reached at about 25 cm from the anal verge (AV). This shortening operation is the most important part of colonoscope insertion.

Pattern A: Even after passing through the bend from the rectosigmoid (Rs) to the sigmoid colon, the intestinal tract lumen observed on the monitor looks like it is running continuously rightward. Therefore, the endoscopist can reach the descending colon without worrying about the SD junction simply by repeatedly rotating the scope clockwise with the right hand.

However, despite its ease and simplicity, you will still need to be careful when using this method as repeated clockwise rotations tend to form an α-loop. To prevent this, it is important to offset the twist of the scope (to maintain the scope's axis in the correct condition) every time you pass through a bend using a clockwise rotation.

Pattern B: After Rs has been passed, the intestinal tract lumen observed on the monitor looks like it is running continuously to the left. In this case, the sigmoid colon is slightly longer than usual. Here, the endoscopist must shift the sigmoid colon so that it is running to the right, instead of left. Otherwise, advancing the scope is likely to result in the formation of an α-loop.

The first opportunity for rightward development is during insertion from Rs into the sigmoid colon. If it is not possible there, insert the scope a little further, catch a bend and try shifting to the right again. The trick here is to capture a fold in a bend in the same way as the hooking-the-fold technique and rotating the scope clockwise.

Once the sigmoid colon is shifted to the right, advance the scope to the right as in Pattern A until it enters the descending colon. The timing of the rightward shift is the most important point when inserting into a Pattern B sigmoid colon. If this maneuver is not possible, ignore the α-loop, that forms and advance the scope to the SD junction. Then, cancel the loop at 40 to 50 cm from AV.

If the scope is pulled carelessly while eliminating the loop, the distal end will immediately slip back as far as Rs. To prevent this, the scope should be pulled slowly without changing the position of the distal end, while searching for right point to cancel the loop with the angulating operation of the left hand and the rotating operation of the right hand. Loops can usually be eliminated easily using angulation and clockwise rotation of the scope if the configuration of the sigmoid colon is uncomplicated, but are more difficult to eliminate when it is complex.

Pattern C: This will be discussed in the discussion of colonic elongation cases (page 171).

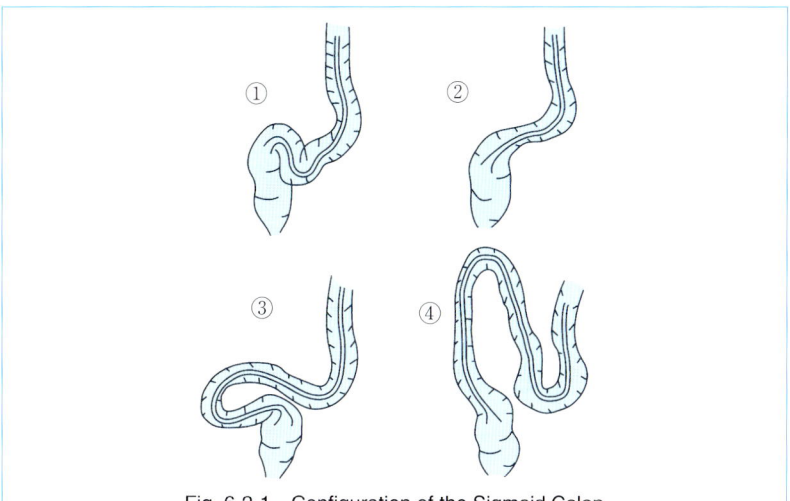

Fig. 6-2-1   Configuration of the Sigmoid Colon
① and ② correspond to Pattern A in which the intestinal tract is oriented toward the left, while its monitor image shows it running continuously rightward. ③ corresponds to Pattern B, in which the intestinal tract develops toward the right while its monitor image shows it running to the left. ④ corresponds to Pattern C, in which the intestinal tract extends to a point near the diaphragm in the abdominal cavity.

③ There are two ways to pass SD: the push method and the pull method

Masahiro Igarashi

1. Push method

This method passes SD by pushing the scope forward, without worrying about the formation of loops. As shown in **Fig. 6-3-1**, the SD junction can be passed by pushing the scope without canceling the $α$-loop or reverse $α$-loop that forms in the sigmoid colon.

However, as this method involves some discomfort for the patient, it is essential to straighten the scope as soon as you have passed SD in order to minimize the patient discomfort.

2. Pull method

The basic technique of this method is the right-turn shortening. After hooking the bend with the distal end, pull the scope while turning its shaft clockwise. This passes the scope through the bend, while straightening

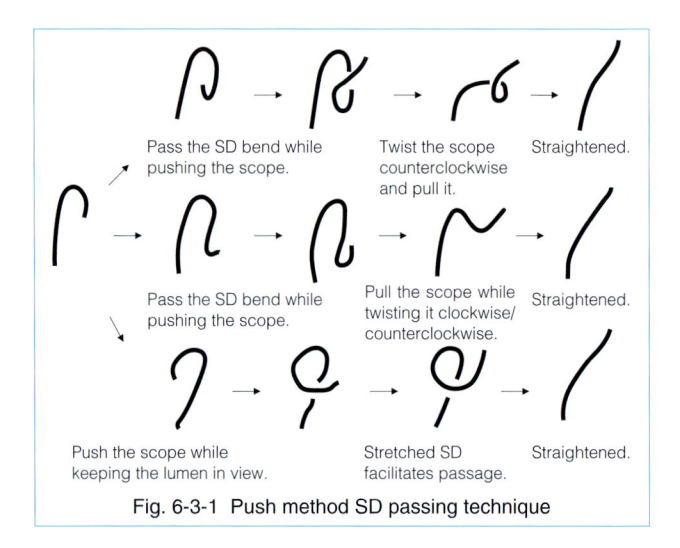

Pass the SD bend while pushing the scope.
Twist the scope counterclockwise and pull it.
Straightened.

Pass the SD bend while pushing the scope.
Pull the scope while twisting it clockwise/counterclockwise.
Straightened.

Push the scope while keeping the lumen in view.
Stretched SD facilitates passage.
Straightened.

Fig. 6-3-1 Push method SD passing technique

Right-turn shortening.

After advancing and withdrawing the scope, pull it when it has passed the bend. Repeat this procedure, inserting the scope as if pressing down on the bend.

If a loop forms, withdraw the scope to make SD as straight as possible, and then insert the scope as if dragging the fold toward you.

Fig. 6-3-2　Pull method SD passing technique

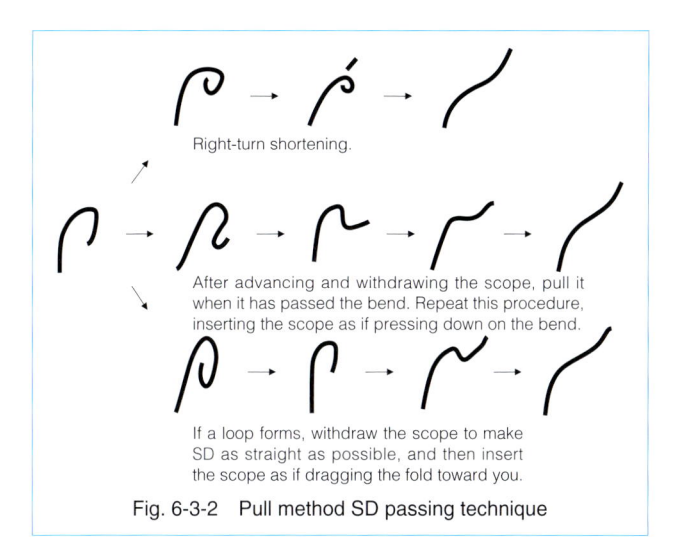

the scope. However, this method is not applicable to every case.

If a loop is formed as shown in **Fig. 6-3-2**, pull the scope as far as possible and cancel or reduce the loop. It is acceptable if a loop of some extent is present before passing the SD junction. After passing through the SD bend by pushing the scope, pull the scope by gently twisting it clockwise or counterclockwise. The effective twisting direction is the direction advancing the distal end. After confirming the effective direction, pull the scope gently while twisting in that direction. When the distal end starts to advance briskly as if it is springing up toward the oral side during pulling, fix the shaft, angulate the scope and maintain the lumen. This causes the distal end to advance and pass through the SD junction at the same time as the scope is straightened. As this method requires a higher degree of skill, it should only be tried by endoscopists who are able to use the push method to pass SD quickly.

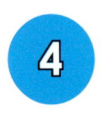

④ Shortening and stretching techniques for the sigmoid colon

Toru Mitsushima

Ultimately, when looking at the various techniques used to pass through the SD junction, it all comes down to two basic techniques: the shortening technique in which the sigmoid colon is barely stretched and no loops are formed; and the stretching technique in which loops of various sizes are formed.

1. Sigmoid colon shortening technique

When the sigmoid colon is short and free of convoluted bends, you can easily advance the scope to the descending colon without really noticing the SD bend simply by using the hooking-the-fold technique[※] described in "Passing the Rs-S Junction" in Chapter 5 (page 64).

This technique is the easiest way to get past the SD and causes the least discomfort, so the patient has very little sense of abdominal distension. On the downside, however, this technique does not facilitate adequate observation during scope insertion because the mucosa of the sigmoid colon is not stretched enough.

When performing colonoscopies using a thin colonoscope, I use the sigmoid colon shortening technique about 30% of the time.

2. Sigmoid colon stretching technique

With the sigmoid colon stretching technique, both the scope and the sigmoid colon form loops during SD passage. There are two main types of loop formed with this technique: the α-loop, where both the scope and sigmoid colon form counterclockwise loops; and the compound loop, in which the scope forms a clockwise loop and the sigmoid colon forms a counterclockwise loop. There are also a number of loops that cannot be classified.

※ Shinya, H.: Colonoscopy, Diagnosis and Treatment of Colonic Disease. Igakushoin, Tokyo, 1982

① α-loop: When the sigmoid colon is relatively short, both the scope and sigmoid colon often form counterclockwise loops, and there are two patterns as follows. With the small α-loop, the twisting of the scope and the looping of the intestinal tract can be stretched by rotating the scope by 180° clockwise (single right turn). With the big α-loop formed when the sigmoid colon is longer or has an adhesion, both the scope and sigmoid colon form big counterclockwise loops, which cannot be stretched with a single (180°) right-turn shortening technique but require an additional rotation (double right turns). The "α-turn" technique[※], a two-person technique developed by Tajima, is similar to the big α-loop stretching technique.

Next to the sigmoid colon shortening technique, the small α-loop technique causes the least amount of discomfort to the patient. The big α-loop stretching technique, on the other hand, must be performed more carefully as it involves a risk that the patient will experience a strong sense of abdominal distension.

② **Compound loops**: In general, when performing colonoscopies on Japanese patients who often have long sigmoid colons, loop formation in opposite directions (compound loops) — in which the scope forms a clockwise loop because of strong clockwise twisting, while the sigmoid colon forms a counterclockwise loop due to its own rotation and warping — tends to occur quite frequently (about 50% of the cases I have handled).

These loops cannot be dissolved with the simple right-turn shortening technique. Instead, slowly rotate the scope 90° counterclockwise to untwist it, and then rotate it clockwise to remove the loop in the sigmoid colon (left- and right-turn shortening technique). I may be the first who pointed out this fact. As with the big α-loop, there is a risk that the patient may experience pain or abdominal distension, so it is important to be extra careful when performing the scope maneuver to remove compound loops.

※ 田島　強，他：Colonoscopy について．Gastroenterol. Endosc 12: 221-222, 1970

⑤ Methods for passing through the sigmoid colon

Masao Ando

The method for crossing the SD junction depends on how the sigmoid colon is passed.

1. Non-push technique

This technique passes folds carefully by combining angulation control using the left hand, rotation, pullback and suction control with the right hand, and hand pressure on the abdomen. Insufflation should be avoided to the extent possible, and the scope push operation that would stretch the intestinal tract is avoided altogether.

When the scope is inserted into the SD junction, a gentle clockwise torque force is usually applied. For details on hand pressure during this procedure, refer to Chapter 2, "Changing the Patient's Position and Applying Hand Pressure" (page 19).

2. Push technique

If, after several retries, the scope still cannot be advanced with the non-push technique, then it becomes necessary to use the push operation to stretch the intestinal tract. Care must be taken, however, because pushing the scope blindly can cause the patient pain and make subsequent advancement difficult. First try pushing slowly and gently to check the resistance felt by the right hand, the distance the scope advances and how the endoscopic view field develops. Angulate and rotate the scope to find the orientation with the least resistance and twisting.

Once the basic orientation is determined, continue inserting the scope by repeating the cycle of small push and pause. Never push the scope continuously for a long period. Naturally, you will need to fine-tune the orientation during advancement. With the push technique, there are cases in which insertion all the way to the splenic flexure is possible with a single straightening of the stretched intestinal tract, while in other cases, the same maneuver has to be repeated several times.

1) Push-once type

If a series of push operations stalls due to an acute bend, it usually occurs at the SD junction. In this case, the right-turn shortening technique is often used. I will not go into the details here — interested readers are encouraged to refer to other literature focusing on this technique — but my impression is that this technique is hard to practice when the scope is inserted with the patient in the supine position.

In such a case, I insert the scope's distal end into the descending colon by angulating it upward and then pull the scope slowly while deaerating the air. While pulling the scope, rotate it in the direction so that the distal end does not come out, which is usually the counterclockwise direction. When the scope is angulated upward, the lumen is basically invisible but the monitor image is not completely red. The scope should feel as if it is sliding smoothly on the mucosal surface. If it does not feel smooth, it is necessary to return and retry. Strong resistance should never be felt. Return and retry is necessary even before any resistance is felt.

Insertion as far as the splenic flexure is sometimes possible with a series of push operations without encountering stalling or resistance. The technique used here seems to be what is called the "α-loop" technique. There are cases where this technique is easiest for insertion and those where insertion is difficult unless this technique is used. Some endoscopists select this technique first, but I usually turn to it as a last resort.

2) Push-again type

With difficult cases, it is necessary to repeat the push and straighten operations. Insert the scope slowly, being careful not to insufflate excessive air, while being alert to any signs of discomfort from the patient.

6 The SD junction is the best and most important part for the "straightening and shortening method" of insertion

Hiroshi Kashida

1. Start shortening the sigmoid colon immediately after entering it

To pass through the sigmoid colon, you should use the shortening technique repeatedly right from the beginning to keep it straight. When the scope's distal end enters the sigmoid colon, angulate the scope slightly upward and advance it little by little while rotating it clockwise (right-turn shortening). Advance the scope by sliding it along the mucosa, rather than pushing it. A big fold can be hooked with the scope tip and pulled to fold the intestine, thereby advancing the scope (hooking-the-fold technique).

By repeating this technique, the sigmoid colon can be folded and shortened in a shape that resembles a wrung-out towel. If the sigmoid colon is short, you will go right past the SD junction while hardly noticing it, simply by repeating the above-mentioned procedure, with an insertion length of 25 to 30 cm (**Fig. 6-6-1**).

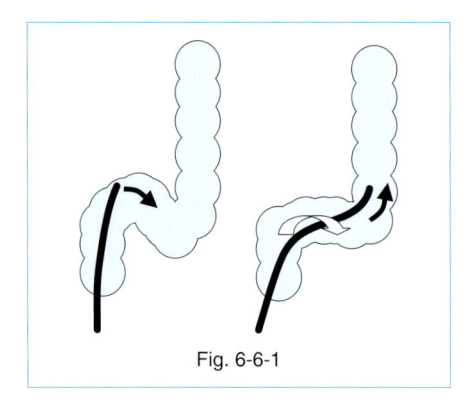

Fig. 6-6-1

Fig. 6-6-2

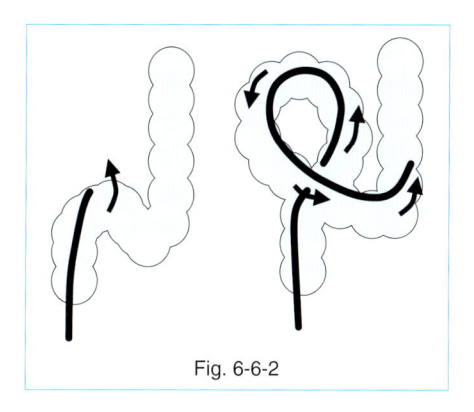

2. If the lumen appears on the left of the monitor image

When the sigmoid colon is nearly straight, the lumen will normally be visible in the right of the monitor image. In some cases, however, the lumen actually continues to appear on the left, even if you try to twist the scope clockwise. If the scope is pushed in such cases, the sigmoid colon forms a so-called α-loop (**Fig. 6-6-2**). Such a loop can be resolved after the scope reaches the descending colon by twisting the scope clockwise and pulling it back substantially (this operation is sometimes called the right-turn shortening).

However, as resolving a loop after it has been formed can cause the patient a fair amount of pain, it is a good idea to try not to form a loop in the first place. Always be aware of the insertion length. If it reaches 40 cm before the scope reaches the SD junction, you can assume that the intestinal tract is already stretched and needs to be shortened before it would be stretched further.

3. Shortening at the S-top

When the colon is long or shortening is insufficient, the sigmoid colon is stretched toward the cranial side and its central section is bent significantly, forming a so-called "S-top". The trick here is to hook a fold of the bend gently with the scope and pull it back using a clockwise twisting

Fig. 6-6-3

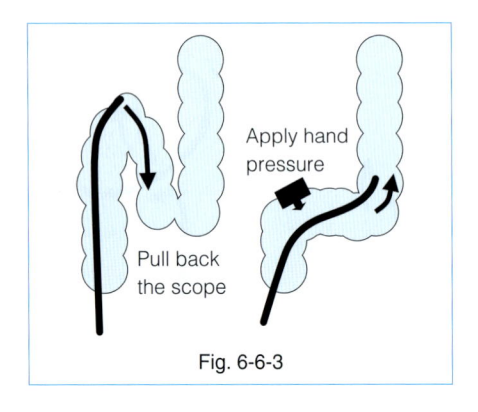

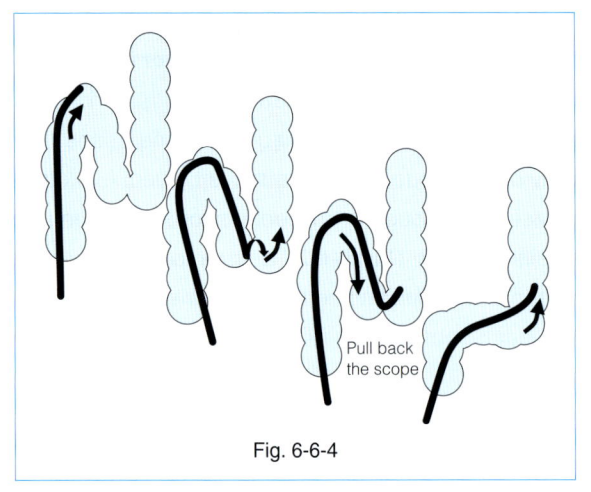

Fig. 6-6-4

motion (**Fig. 6-6-3**).

If passage is difficult, change the patient position from the left lateral to the supine position, or have the assistant apply hand pressure from the cranial side toward the caudal side. If the S-top is passed by just pushing the scope without shortening, a loop called an N-loop tends to be formed (**Fig. 6-6-4**).

4. If the SD junction is acute

The angle of the SD junction gets more acute when the sigmoid colon is more stretched. To shorten the sigmoid colon, the scope should be pulled with a clockwise twisting motion at a point before the SD junction. Sometimes, however, the scope slips back during your effort of shortening the colon and pushing it once more also stretches the colon again. In such a case, have the assistant apply hand pressure from the right to the left before pushing the scope. Insertion of the scope is easier with the patient in the supine or right lateral position, rather than the left lateral position.

Once the sigmoid colon has been shortened successfully, angulate the scope upward and pull it a little with a clockwise twisting motion so that the distal end enters the descending colon. If the sigmoid colon cannot be shortened, angulating the scope sharply upward and twisting it clockwise at the SD junction sometimes makes it possible to insert only the distal end of the scope into the descending colon. Then, pull back he scope slowly to shorten the sigmoid colon, taking care not to let the scope tip slip off (**Fig. 6-6-4**). Once the sigmoid colon is shortened adequately, resistance felt by the right hand should almost disappear.

7. Passing the Splenic Flexure

How to deal with problems at the splenic flexure

Shinji Tanaka

1. Getting from the splenic flexure to the transverse colon

Typically, the endoscopist will barely be aware of the splenic flexure during colonoscopic insertion. You will know you are there when the transverse colon (typical triangular intestinal lumen accompanied by clear folds) comes into view.

The usual way to advance the scope from the splenic flexure to the transverse colon is to suction air in the left part of the transverse colon as much as possible, shorten the tract and smooth out the bend. This keeps the distance the scope has to travel to a minimum so you can pass the middle part of the transverse colon easily. As you are doing this, it is critical to rotate slightly clockwise the scope so that it does not warp.

2. If you have trouble passing the splenic flexure

Usually, you should have no trouble passing the splenic flexure; however, in some cases, passage is difficult even when the sigmoid colon has almost been straightened. If this happens, hand compression may help prevent the sigmoid colon from deflecting, but changing the patient's position is often more effective than hand compression.

If a problem is encountered in passage of the splenic flexure while the patient is in the left lateral position, the first thing to do is change the patient to the supine position. This moves the air inside the colon and makes it more difficult for the sigmoid colon to deflect, facilitating insertion into the transverse colon.

If this position change does not work, try changing to the right lateral position. In most cases, insertion from the splenic flexure to the transverse colon is quite easy when the patient is in the right lateral position. If insertion is still difficult even after changing the patient's position, use hand compression on the abdomen as well.

② Splenic flexure bending toward the left

Satoru Tamura

After the scope has crossed the SD junction through the application of shortening and straightening techniques, it extends from the descending colon to the splenic flexure, reaching a point about 40 cm from the anal verge. Since the splenic flexure is a bending section where the descending colon shifts direction toward the anterior wall and reaches the transverse colon, it can be recognized in endoscopic observation as a fold bending toward the left (**Fig. 7-2-1**).

To pass the splenic flexure and enter the transverse colon, suction air to minimize the bend, catch the bend with the scope's distal end, rotate the scope counterclockwise and push it gently, being careful not to twist the sigmoid colon. If the bend is too acute to allow you to advance the scope, changing the patient's position (right lateral position) is usually effective.

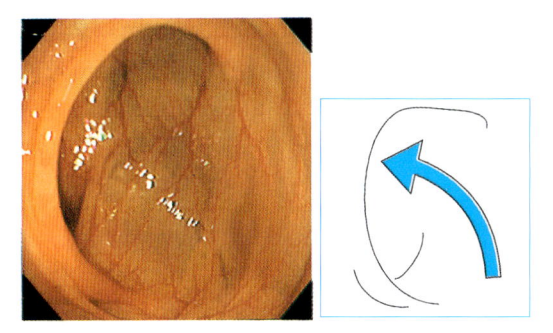

Fig. 7-2-1 Splenic flexure bending toward the left

③ Tips for smooth passage of the splenic flexure

Norihiro Hamamoto

1. Novices have problems with previous methods

After suctioning enough air out of the descending colon to flatten out the bend at the splenic flexure as much as possible, you will be able to obtain a view of the left part of the transverse colon by rotating the scope counterclockwise. The transverse colon's lumen has a triangular shape formed by three colic teniae, so it is relatively easy to recognize. Before continuing, make sure you straighten the scope. If the scope is straightened, the splenic flexure should be reached from the descending colon at about 40 cm from the anal canal.

The transverse colon is approached with the patient in the left lateral or supine position. I put the patient in the supine position after the S-top, so am able to approach the transverse colon without changing the patient position. While viewing the center of the lumen from the front, push the scope forward, while angulating it downward. In most cases, the scope will pass through the splenic flexure and reach the middle part of the transverse colon.

Of course, it is not unusual for passage to be difficult; however, with novices, problems are often caused by improper insertion to the descending colon. If too much air is insufflated into the sigmoid colon, loops tend to re-form easily even after the colon has been straightened. Care is required in the approaches to the descending colon, sigmoid colon and rectum; whether or not they are performed correctly will determine the ease of subsequent insertion maneuvers.

2. What to do when passage is difficult

With slender female patients with acute splenic flexure bending, patients with dolichosigmoid, or patients with adhesion after laparotomy, the scope can easily get warped in the sigmoid colon or cannot be advanced but simply keeps bumping up against the left diaphragm no matter hard it is pushed.

To prevent warping in such a case, push the scope by applying gently slight clockwise rotation so as not to twist the sigmoid colon. In addition, placing the patient in the right lateral position allows the transverse colon's own weight to straighten it out. Suctioning air collected between the splenic flexure and the left part of the transverse colon makes the splenic flexure angle less acute, also facilitating insertion.

Application of hand pressure from the upper right point of the umbilicus toward the left groin or from the abdomen or back side of the left hypochondrium is also recommended, as this may prevent re-looping of the sigmoid colon. Deep breathing can also be effective sometimes.

The Variable Stiffness scope is a useful modality for approaching the splenic flexure because its shaft can be set to be more pliable until the passage around the SD junction and then set to be more rigid after the splenic flexure is reached. Insertion into the splenic flexure can be especially difficult if a slim scope is used.

If hand pressure and changing the patient position prove ineffective, a sliding tube should be inserted. If the sliding tube is not already attached, withdraw the scope quickly, attach a sliding tube and retry insertion. This is the quickest way to pass the splenic flexure.

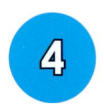

④ How to achieve smooth insertion into splenic flexure

Yuji Inoue

1. Before insertion into splenic flexure

The rectum, descending colon and ascending colon are fixed, while the sigmoid colon and transverse colon are mobile. Generally, insertion of a colonoscope is easy from a fixed region to mobile region of the colon.

This applies specifically to the passage from the rectum to the sigmoid colon and from the descending colon to the transverse colon (splenic flexure). Smooth insertion can be assured by keeping certain points in mind. In this section, I will discuss those points relevant to passage of the splenic flexure.

2. How to insert the scope into the splenic flexure

1) Try shortening the sigmoid colon before insertion into the splenic flexure:

It is essential that the sigmoid colon has been shortened and the scope straightened before insertion into the splenic flexure. Inserting the scope into the descending colon using the shortening technique of folding the sigmoid colon facilitates painless colonoscopic insertion without using a sedative or analgesic I have been proposing.

If the scope is inserted into the descending colon when a loop has formed in the sigmoid colon, the sigmoid colon should be shortened with the scope as soon as it has been inserted into the descending colon. After insertion into the descending colon, jiggle the scope around and confirm that the scope can follow the colon and that the intestinal tract is shortened (the actual distance of the scope from the anal verge is less than 40 cm).

Even when the scope is inserted almost perfectly, a small loop could form and deeper insertion would stretch the sigmoid colon excessively. In this case, try shortening the colon by jiggling the scope while applying clockwise torque. If the loop is still there, use hand pressure. The trick to hand pressure is to apply it so that simple compression of the abdomen can move the scope into the oral side of the descending colon. Once you get used to it, you will be able to feel the compression with the right hand even when the scope is kept stationary.

2) Insertion into splenic flexure (to the entrance of transverse colon)

Once the scope is in the proximity of the splenic flexure, insert it into the entrance of the transverse colon using rotation only — never push the scope. Advancing the scope from the splenic flexure to the middle part of the transverse colon is mainly based on pushing, but insertion from the splenic flexure to the transverse colon should be done using the rotation operation (as if "hooking" the transverse colon).

At this time, rotate the scope clockwise and insert it into the entrance of the transverse colon while attempting shortening. This makes it possible to shorten the left-side colon completely (about 40 cm from the anal verge). Use care not to insert the scope into the transverse colon by pushing, as this may cause the "walking stick phenomenon" that hinders insertion into the deeper region.

Fluoroscopic observation of the splenic flexure using contrast enema sometimes detects a large number of bends in this region. With such cases, every fold should be passed carefully as you would in insertion into the sigmoid colon. If an external loop (an extracorporeal loop) forms, eliminate it to avoid problems with the subsequent insertion (**Fig. 7-4-1**).

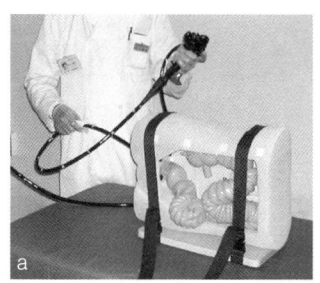

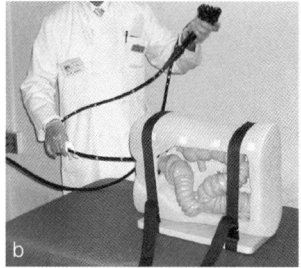

Fig. 7-4-1

3) Insertion from the splenic flexure to the middle part of transverse colon

When advancing the scope from the transverse colon to the cecum, you should mainly use the push operation; however, it is recommended that you do not forget to keep an eye open for opportunities for shortening during insertion. If the lumen is viewed from the front, the scope angle becomes acute as shown in **Fig. 7-4-2a**, making it hard to transmit force to the deeper region.

To facilitate the transmission of force to the deeper region, it is recommended to insert while looking at the upper part of the transverse colon as shown in **Fig. 7-4-2b**. If a loop forms in the sigmoid colon, use hand pressure. If you are using a scope with Variable Stiffness, increase the stiffness. Deep breathing can also be effective sometimes. If none of these measures is effective, setting the patient in the right lateral position may make insertion possible, as discussed previously in the description of the patient position change.

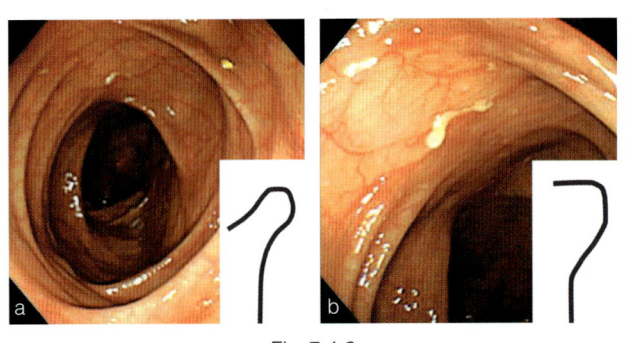

Fig. 7-4-2

5 Importance of straightening the scope and making the splenic flexure less acute

Osamu Tsuruta, Hiroshi Kawano

To ensure smooth, reliable passage through the splenic flexure, several key points need to be kept in mind, regarding both scope status before passage and scope maneuvering during passage.

1. Status before splenic flexure passage (straightening of the scope)
To pass through the splenic flexure properly, the scope should be straightened so that the pushing force can be effectively transmitted to the distal end. To confirm that the scope is straight before splenic flexure passage, check the following:
1) The distance from the anal verge should be around 40 cm.
2) Move the scope gently forwards and backwards and confirm that the movement of the distal end on the monitor screen is sufficiently

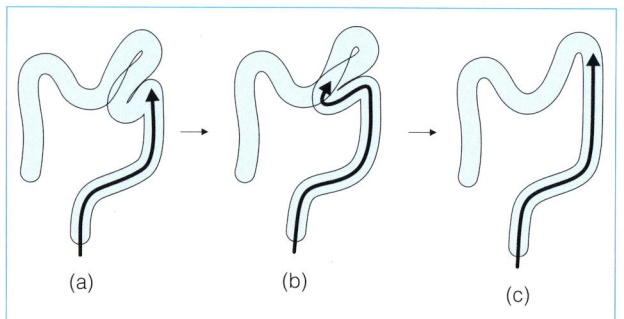

(a) (b) (c)

Fig. 7-5-1 Case in which a bend on the oral side of the descending colon makes it difficult for the scope to reach the splenic flexure
a) The bend is sometimes mistaken for the splenic flexure.
b) Insert the distal end to the oral side of the bend by pushing the scope.
c) Remove the loop while pulling the scope so that the scope is straight when it reaches the splenic flexure.

synchronized with the scope movement.

3) Remove your right hand from the scope and confirm that the scope's distal end does not slip back.

Even when conditions 1) to 3) are met, the scope may not reach the splenic flexure if the intestinal tract is bent on the oral side of the descending colon (**Fig. 7-5-1a**). In this case, insert the distal end as far as the oral side of the bend by pushing the scope (**Fig. 7-5-1b**) and then remove the loop while pulling the scope so that the scope reaches the splenic flexure in the straightened condition (**Fig. 7-5-1c**).

2. During splenic flexure passage

1) Methods for preventing loop formation in the sigmoid colon

a) Apply torque

While twisting the scope clockwise, set the Variable Stiffness slightly stiffer

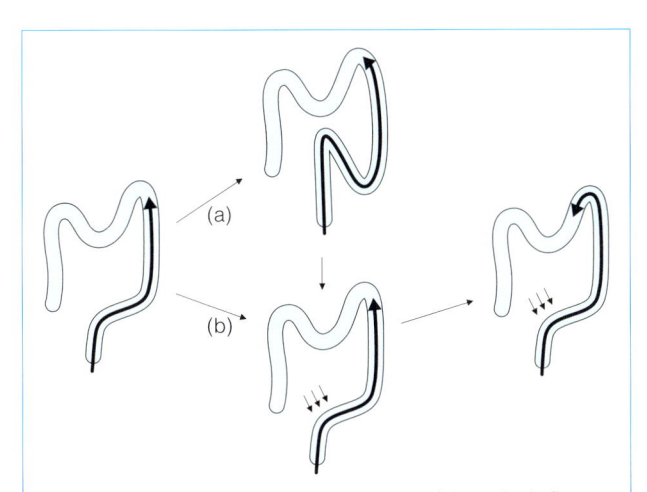

Fig. 7-5-2 Hand pressure when passage of the splenic flexure passage is difficult
a) If a loop forms in the sigmoid colon, it may not be possible to advance scope to the oral side.
b) Hand pressure is recommended to prevent the sigmoid colon from stretching.

and advance the scope to prevent formation of a loop in the sigmoid colon.

b) Apply hand pressure (**Fig. 7-5-2**)

If method a) cannot advance the scope to the oral side due to loop formation, it is recommended to apply hand pressure to prevent the sigmoid colon from stretching.

2) Methods for making the splenic flexure less acute

a) Downward angulation

When the transverse colon lumen comes into view, angulate the scope downward and advance it little by little toward the oral side. The downward angulation will reduce the bend in the splenic flexure and facilitate the passage.

b) Deep breathing

Have the patient breath in and hold their breath. The lowering of the diaphragm presses the scope from the head direction and minimizes the bend at the splenic flexure.

c) Patient position change

If none of the methods described in a) and b) above allows passage of the splenic flexure, try changing the patient position — to the supine position if the current position is left lateral, and to the right lateral position if passage is still impossible in the supine position. Changing the position can also help make the splenic flexure less acute.

6 What you need to know about splenic flexure passage

Yusuke Saitoh

Important points

- If the scope length at the splenic flexure is longer than 40 to 45 cm, remove the loop in the sigmoid colon before advancing into the transverse colon.
- During insertion, attenuate the angulation slightly and apply a slightly clockwise rotation.
- Combine hand pressure and/or patient position change. Using the right lateral position and suctioning air are the most effective ways to facilitate insertion.

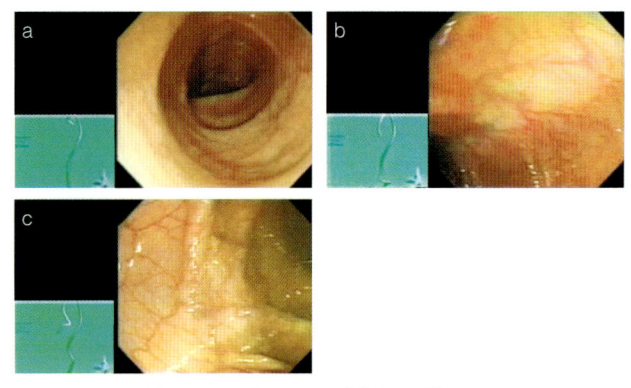

Fig. 7-6-1 Passage of Splenic Flexure
a) The scope length at the splenic flexure should be 40 to 45 cm. If the insertion length is longer, remove the loop of the sigmoid colon before insertion into the transverse colon.
b) To insert the scope into the transverse colon, twist the scope lightly clockwise, attenuate the angle of upward angulation and insert the scope as if it is sliding along the colon wall. Also apply hand pressure to the sigmoid colon.
c) The scope can be inserted as far as the middle part of the transverse colon.

- If the bend is acute, use the hooking-the-fold technique.

Assuming the scope is straight, the length to the splenic flexure in Japanese people is 40 to 45 cm. If the scope length is longer than this when the triangular lumen corresponding to the transverse colon comes in to view (**Fig. 7-6-1a**), a loop may form in the sigmoid colon so the scope will have to be straightened. You can confirm that the scope is straight by moving it slightly back and forth and confirming that the distal end moves in synch (one-to-one movement).

It is easy to identify when a loop has formed because the loop interferes with the transmission of subtle hand movements to the distal end. Be sure to remove the sigmoid colon loop before proceeding with insertion into the transverse colon.

When inserting the scope into the transverse colon, rotate the scope slightly clockwise and push to attenuate the angulation slightly for smooth insertion. During insertion, do not orient the scope toward the center of the lumen of the left part of the transverse colon; instead, advance it along the colon wall in the direction of the attenuated angulation (**Fig. 7-6-1b**).

If the patient is a slender woman with a long transverse colon, you must take care to avoid formation of a γ-loop in the transverse colon. If a loop forms again in the sigmoid colon, try hand pressure (abdominal manipulation) a little below and from the right of the umbilicus. You can also apply pressure to the area above and to the left of the umbilicus.

If hand pressure (abdominal manipulation) alone fails to prevent the loop from being re-formed, turn the patient to the right lateral position, suction out excess air and retry insertion. Changing the patient position is effective in dealing with insertion difficulty in any region. In some cases, splenic flexures may have several bends. These bends should be passed using the hooking-the-fold technique, in the same way as when passing through the sigmoid colon (**Fig. 7-6-1c**).

8. Advancing in the Transverse Colon

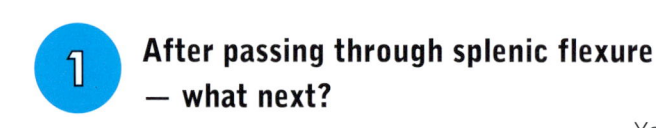

① After passing through splenic flexure — what next?

Yasumoto Suzuki

1. Before advancing into the transverse colon

The insertion methods used for the anal side and oral side of the splenic flexure differ quite significantly. This is because of the difference in the way that force is transmitted to the scope's distal end before and after the splenic flexure.

On the anal side, force is transmitted more effectively on the splenic flexure, so you can advance the scope without being concerned about force transmission. However, once the splenic flexure has been passed, less force is transmitted, so you will need to use an insertion method that will not reduce the transmitted force.

2. After passing the splenic flexure

After the splenic flexure has been passed, the left part of the transverse colon comes into view. However, if you try to push the scope toward the lumen using a counterclockwise rotation, the scope will not advance because the amount of force transmitted to the distal end decreases.

In this case, the scope should be pushed with a light clockwise rotation toward the 2 o'clock direction of the lumen. This makes it possible to advance the scope while ensuring that a sufficient amount of force is transmitted to the scope's distal end.

As the scope is pushed with a slight clockwise rotation, the lumen appears in the bottom left of the monitor image. Angulate the scope (usually downward) so that the lumen is visible in the center, and push the scope again with a light clockwise rotation. Repeating the rightward rotation and downward angulation will advance the scope to the middle part of the transverse colon.

3. When the middle section of the transverse colon comes into view

As you advance the scope through the left part of the transverse colon, you will encounter an acute leftward (or downward) bend (**Fig. 8-1-1**). This is the bend in the middle part of the transverse colon. To pass through here, always push the scope using counterclockwise rotation, while angling it upwards.

Once the bend in the middle part of the transverse colon has been passed and the right side of the transverse colon comes clearly into view, pull the scope using counterclockwise rotation combined with upward angulation to shorten the transverse colon so that the bend of the hepatic flexure in the deeper part of the colon (**Fig. 8-1-2**) is visible in the bottom right on the proximal side of the image (**Fig. 8-1-3**). If this procedure is done properly, it is not difficult to pass through the hepatic flexure.

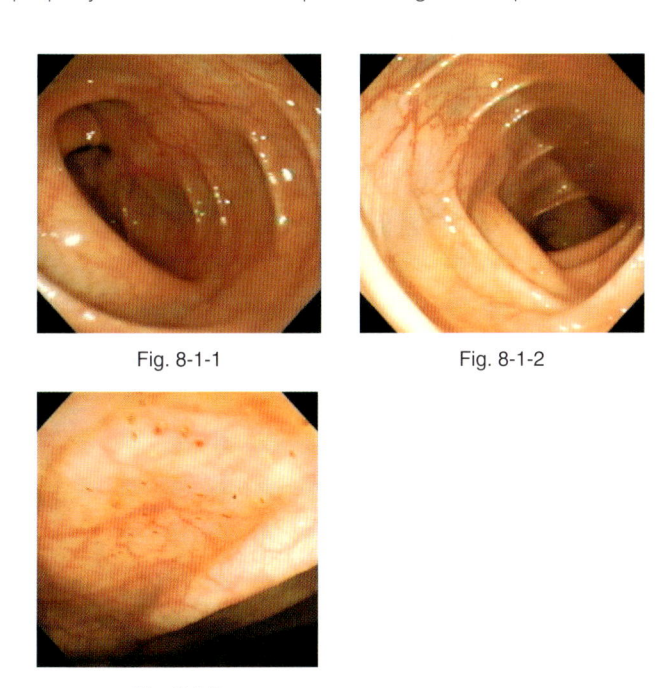

Fig. 8-1-1

Fig. 8-1-2

Fig. 8-1-3

② Suction and intestinal tract shortening are also essential in the transverse colon

Norihiro Hamamoto

1. Maneuvering in the transverse colon mainly involves counterclockwise rotation

As well as being easier to pass through, it is easier to keep the scope on the luminal axis in the lumen of the transverse colon than it is in other regions. Nevertheless, you will still need to be careful; if you push the scope through the transverse colon improperly, you will end up having trouble with subsequent insertion from the hepatic flexure to the ascending colon.

For smooth passage through the transverse colon, it is important to approach it from the splenic flexure after shortening and straightening the segment up to the descending colon. Unlike other regions, the main maneuver here is the counterclockwise rotation of the scope. After you pass the splenic flexure and reach the bend in the middle part of the transverse colon, you will find that the subsequent intestinal tract in most cases extends toward the left.

Now, rotate the scope counterclockwise so that the intestinal tract axis is on the vertical axis of the monitor image, angulate the scope upward to hook a fold with the distal end, and pull back the scope while twisting it counterclockwise to enter the right part of the transverse colon. This lumen can be found easily by applying suction little by little to relax the intestinal tract. If the lumen is hard to find because the bend in the middle of the transverse colon is acute, angulate the scope upward, pull it back a little, and repeat light pushing operations while twisting the scope in both directions.

In general, the supine position is recommended for the approach after reaching the splenic flexure. You can leave the patient in this position until you reach the middle part of the transverse colon. At this point, if the lumen of the right part of the transverse colon has collapsed and is hard to find, put the patient back in the left lateral position. This will widen the lumen and facilitate insertion.

2. Suction brings the hepatic flexure closer

After inserting the scope in the right part of the transverse colon, twist the scope counterclockwise and pull it as if tucking it up toward the abdomen. This causes the scope to advance (paradoxical movement) and reach the hepatic flexure. Usually, just suctioning air will bring the hepatic flexure closer in this process, but it is recommended that you also angulate the scope to keep the center of the lumen in sight.

If you have trouble at all shortening the transverse colon, push the scope until the hepatic flexure. If a γ-loop forms, you may still be able to pass the scope through the hepatic flexure easily and reach the cecum without causing any pain. On the other hand, if the patient complains of pain, twist the scope counterclockwise to readjust the lumen or withdraw the scope to the splenic flexure and retry insertion.

After the hepatic flexure, the lumen extends in the 3 o'clock direction in most cases, so rotating the scope clockwise usually allows it to reach the ascending colon. Although it is often necessary to change the patient position in the transverse colon (excluding the splenic and hepatic flexures), hand pressure is not usually required in this region. However, when the transverse colon is long and droops, it can be helpful to apply pressure between the umbilicus area and the suprapubic area.

In the approach to the transverse colon, too, insufflating too much air in the section leading to the splenic flexure or excessive stretching of the sigmoid colon results in deflection of the sigmoid colon, as well as limiting maneuverability. The same rules that apply to insertion elsewhere are also applicable to the transverse colon, that is, suction as much air as possible to collapse the intestinal tract and advance the scope by trying to shorten the intestinal tract.

③ Basic maneuvers and applied techniques

Masahiro Igarashi

1. Basic maneuver

After passing the splenic flexure, take a look at the lumen and push the scope gently to reach the bend in the mid-transverse colon. Once you reach this point, point the scope's distal end toward the lumen and sharply angulate the scope. This will make it possible to pass through the bend in the mid-transverse colon. As soon as the lumen on the oral side becomes visible, twist the scope shaft in both directions (mainly counterclockwise) and pull it back while suctioning air. This will allow the distal end to advance toward the hepatic flexure.

2. If the transverse colon is long

If the patient has a long transverse colon, the scope may not be able to reach the hepatic flexure, after passing through the bend seemingly in the mid-transverse colon using the maneuver described above. In this case, repeat the basic maneuver (passing through each bend and pulling the scope back after it) to reach the hepatic flexure.

3. If a γ-loop forms in the transverse colon

If you cannot advance the scope's distal end using the basic maneuver in

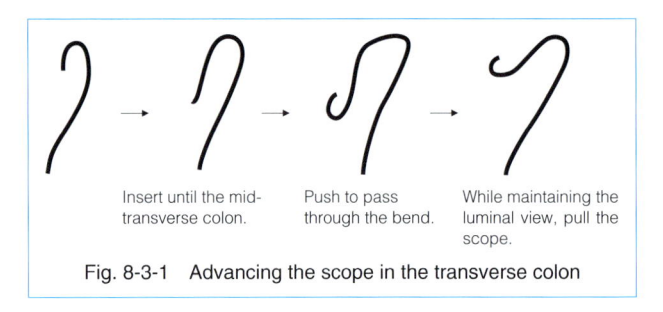

| Insert until the mid-transverse colon. | Push to pass through the bend. | While maintaining the luminal view, pull the scope. |

Fig. 8-3-1   Advancing the scope in the transverse colon

the transverse colon or if the distal end comes out when the scope is pulled back, the only solution is to push the scope. At this time, a γ-loop as shown in **Fig. 8-3-2** may form. If you pull back the scope to straighten it, you may unintentionally withdraw the scope. If this happens, stop pulling the scope and try pushing it instead. Usually, you will be able to advance the scope to the cecum, while the γ-loop in the transverse colon remains in place.

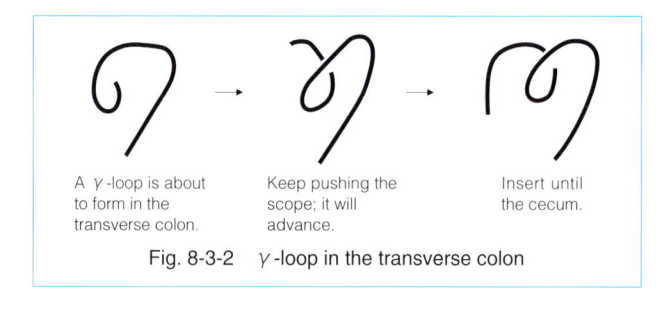

| A γ-loop is about to form in the transverse colon. | Keep pushing the scope; it will advance. | Insert until the cecum. |

Fig. 8-3-2 γ-loop in the transverse colon

④ Key points in passage of transverse colon

Yusuke Saitoh

Key points

- Starting in the left part of the transverse colon, rotate the scope clockwise to advance it to the middle part of the transverse colon.
- Use the hooking-the-fold technique, while rotating the scope counterclockwise, to enter the right part of the transverse colon.
- Together, the "pull-up" operation and suction will advance the scope along the lumen (paradoxical movement) until it reaches the hepatic flexure.

In the middle part of the transverse colon, the subsequent lumen is most often visible in the 6 to 8 o'clock direction (**Fig. 8-4-1a**). By applying

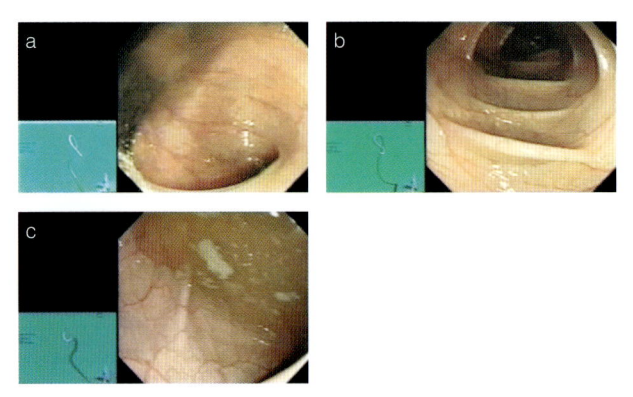

Fig. 8-4-1 How to advance the scope in the transverse colon
a) In the middle part of the transverse colon, the subsequent lumen is most often visible in the 6 to 8 o'clock direction. If this is the case, rotate the scope counterclockwise.
b) Enter the right part of the transverse colon using the hooking-the-fold technique by angulating the scope upward.
c) Pull the scope back along the lumen and suction air to reach the hepatic flexure (paradoxical movement).

counterclockwise rotation while the scope is advancing through the left part of the transverse colon, the scope can be adjusted so that the subsequent lumen is visible in the 11 to 12 o'clock direction when it reaches the middle part of the transverse colon.

After reaching the middle part of the transverse colon, advance toward the right part of the transverse colon by angulating the scope upward and using the hooking-the-fold technique (**Fig. 8-4-1b**). When the lumen comes in view, with enough suction of air, "pull up" the scope (usually while rotating it counterclockwise) to move the scope to the hepatic flexure (paradoxical movement) (**Fig. 8-4-1c**).

Usually, simply rotating the scope clockwise with enough suction of air will advance the scope to the ascending colon. If the patient is thin and has a long transverse colon, a γ-loop may form in the transverse colon, which can be identified when there is an extremely acute bend of the transverse colon or when the scope does not reach the hepatic flexure even when it is pulled back. In this case, remove the loop of the transverse colon (it can be removed by twisting the scope counterclockwise in most cases).

⑤ Tips for advancing the scope in the transverse colon

Hiro-o Yamano

In this section, I am going to discuss the four best ways to advance the scope in the transverse colon and the two basic insertion techniques used.

1. Four tips

1) Tip 1

It is important to have a good understanding of the configuration of the intestinal tract in all three dimensions. The starting point, the splenic flexure, and the end point, the hepatic flexure, are located on the backside. The middle part of the transverse colon sags on the abdomen side, around the umbilicus. It also helps to remember that the contour changes after the peak in the middle part of the transverse colon.

2) Tip 2

The transverse colon is not fixed and can be shortened or straightened. This means that changing the patient position can be an effective way to help advance the scope. On the other hand, it should be noted that this feature also means that there is a high likelihood of excessive stretching and loop formation.

3) Tip 3

After the scope's distal end has reached the splenic flexure, it is important to make sure the scope is straight before advancing it through the transverse colon. Straightening the scope is one of the most basic techniques of endoscopic insertion and is essential to ensure controllability and safety. After reaching the splenic flexure, correct the warping and loops formed in the insertion process up to that point, take a brief pause, and then insert the scope by following its own warping as well as the splenic flexure. Doing this ensures successful insertion.

4) Tip 4

Suction as much air from the lumen as possible. Removing excess air in the splenic and hepatic flexures is especially helpful straightening of the intestinal tract.

2. Two basic insertion techniques

Based on the above-mentioned four tips, there are two basic insertion techniques that can be used to advance the scope in the transverse colon, assuming that the scope has been straightened and is at the splenic flexure side of the transverse colon.

1) Technique 1

This technique consists of simply pushing the scope. The most suitable and least painful patient position for this procedure is the supine or right lateral position rather than the left lateral position.

When the scope's distal end has passed the middle point of the transverse colon, angulate the scope downward so that the distal end points toward the cranial side and then pull back the scope. This maneuver tightens up the transverse colon so that it does not sag. Now you can return the angulation to the neutral position and advance the scope along the right side of the transverse colon to the hepatic flexure.

2) Technique 2

This technique is what is usually referred to "shortening the colonic fold through bending". Angulate the scope upward and rotate it counterclockwise to shorten the intestinal tract and advance from the middle part of the transverse colon to the right part.

This maneuver consists of elevating the scope from the position where the middle part of the transverse colon bends and sags on the abdominal side toward the cranial side, while pushing the transverse colon toward the back. Finally, return the angulation more or less to the neutral direction and rotate the scope clockwise to reach all the way to the hepatic flexure. This technique is possible regardless of the patient position. I usually use the supine position.

Although there are other variations of these techniques, I believe that you can deal with any problem you may encounter by observing these basic tips and insertion techniques.

The importance of shortening the colon and resolving any loops

Hiroshi Kashida

The middle part of the transverse colon is usually bent and sags down, so the insertion method should be somewhat changed at that point. It is helpful to look at the transverse colon as two separate sections: the left half and the right half.

1. From the splenic flexure to the middle part of the transverse colon

If the transverse colon does not have many bends, the triangular lumen will look straight once you have advanced the scope past the splenic flexure. From there, you can easily advance the scope to the middle part of the transverse colon simply by pushing. However, if the sigmoid colon is stretched or has formed a loop while the scope is in the splenic flexure, then pushing the scope will only aggravate the stretching or looping. In such a case, the scope tip does not advance; instead, it may actually slip back (paradoxical movement) and the patient will experience more pain. To prevent this, confirm that the insertion length up to the splenic flexure is

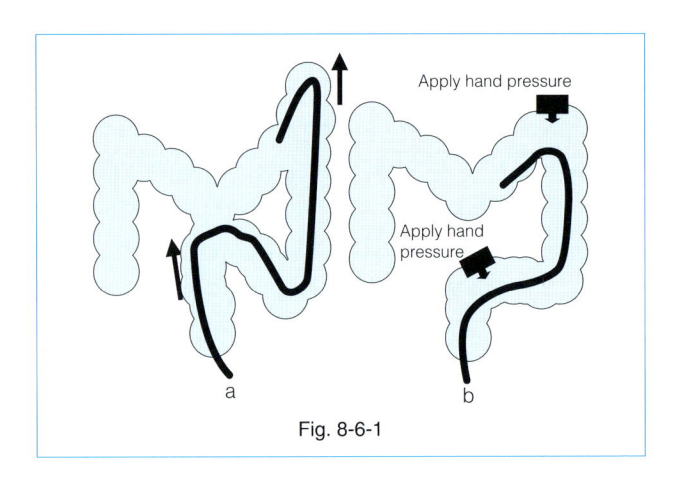

Fig. 8-6-1

about 40 cm. If you feel that the scope has formed any loop, be sure to resolve it (in most cases, this will be possible by pulling back the scope while rotating it clockwise).

If bending of the splenic flexure or sagging of the transverse colon is significant, pushing the scope will cause the bent section near the scope tip to push up the diaphragm (walking-stick phenomenon, shown in **Fig. 8-6-1a**). If this happens, the distal end will not advance, but the sigmoid colon will be stretched and the patient will complain of pain.

In such a case, put the patient in the right lateral position to attenuate the bending angle and facilitate insertion. Hand pressure is also often effective in such a case. Put a finger between the left costal arch and the scope to push down the scope toward the caudal side. With the other hand, press the sigmoid colon from the right to the left so that it does not get stretched (**Fig. 8-6-1b**).

2. From the middle part of transverse colon to the hepatic flexure

When the scope reaches the bend in the middle part of the transverse colon, place the patient in the supine position, angulate the scope upward, hook a fold with it, and pull back the scope while twisting it slightly counterclockwise. This straightens the sagging transverse colon by lifting it toward the cranial side and opens a view of the right part of the

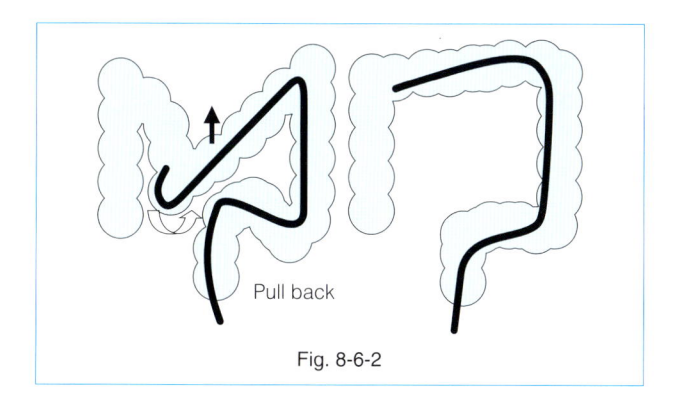

Fig. 8-6-2

transverse colon on the monitor image (**Fig. 8-6-2**). The load imposed on the right hand disappears at the moment the colon is straightened.

If the transverse colon is not straightened, pushing the scope simply aggravates the sagging instead of advancing the scope. Don't keep the patient in the right lateral position because, by doing so, the bend in the middle part of the transverse colon remains acute. Pushing the scope in this condition would easily result in the formation of a γ-loop.

In many cases, another bend may be encountered before the hepatic flexure. Here, too, angulate the scope upward, hook a fold, and pull the scope back while twisting it slightly counterclockwise to advance the scope tip until the hepatic flexure comes into view.

3. The key to success is hidden in the regions before the transverse colon

Passing through the transverse colon is usually not very difficult. However, spending too much time or insufflating too much air during passage of the sigmoid colon or SD junction can stretch the transverse colon, causing problems later. In order to pass through the transverse colon, a stiff scope is better than a pliable scope.

When the transverse colon is long, multiple bends may be encountered one after another. After passing through each bend, pull back the scope, deflate enough amount of air, and fold the intestinal tract toward you. Each bend often appears alternately on the left and right, while, in general, the lumen of the transverse colon extends toward the left of the monitor image.

9. Passing the Hepatic Flexure

1 Remember, "haste makes waste"

Takahisa Matsuda

1. Posture changing (left lateral position) and light manipulation on the right hypochondrium are effective

The reference insertion lengths for a straightened scope (ideal reaching distances) are 20 cm at the S-top, 40 cm at the splenic flexure, 60 cm at the hepatic flexure and 70 to 80 cm at the cecum. Ideally, the movement of the scope's distal end will correspond to the movement of the right hand in a 1:1 relationship without the scope looping or warping. If the scope length matches the reference length for each section of the colon, it means that the scope is straight and distal end movement corresponds to hand movement.

The hepatic flexure is the last bend encountered during a colonoscopy insertion. In most cases, assuming that the scope is inserted straight, the hepatic flexure can be reached at about 60 cm. Whether this region can be passed properly depends on how the scope has been inserted through the transverse colon.

The transverse colon is fixed only loosely by the mesocolon and is highly mobile inside the abdominal cavity. As a result, in the case of an excessively long colon, sagging sometimes makes it difficult for the scope to pass the bend of the hepatic flexure properly.

To avoid sagging and insert the scope into the transverse colon, put the patient in the right lateral position and advance the scope to mid-T by making full use of the up-down slalom technique (while being conscious of maintaining the scope axis).

The reason why the right lateral position is effective is that the non-fixed transverse colon is shifted toward the right by gravity and thus shortened automatically. At the same time, hand pressure on the abdominal wall that pushes the umbilicus upward may also help prevent the transverse colon from sagging.

Usually, after passing mid-T with counterclockwise rotation of the scope, pulling back the scope while twisting it clockwise makes it possible to approach the hepatic flexure. The ideal method for passing the hepatic flexure is to rotate the scope clockwise, while adjusting the air amount so that the scope drops into the ascending colon.

It can also be effective to make use of the variations in the amount of air in the intestinal tract. In other words, the insertion operation can often be facilitated by having the patient take a deep breath and hold it. However, there may also be cases with adhesions after hepatectomy or cholecystectomy or cases with acute bends. With such cases, the patient's posture changing to the left lateral position or light manipulation on the right hypochondrium or the area above the umbilicus may be effective.

2. Always keep in mind that "haste makes waste"

Beginners are often forced to give up insertion in the middle of transverse colon or at the hepatic flexure. This usually happens when they try to pass the hepatic flexure without first having properly corrected any warping or looping of the scope. Retrying insertion while the scope is warped or looped achieves nothing but to inflict more pain on the patient.

In this case, it is likely that the endoscopist will feel that the movement of the hand grasping the scope is restricted. If this happens, it is recommended to suppress the urge to hurry, withdraw the scope temporarily until near the splenic flexure (or sometimes the sigmoid colon) and retry insertion from there. In many circumstances, re-inserting the scope in the properly shortened status makes it very easy to pass through the hepatic flexure.

2 Hepatic flexure bending toward the right

Satoru Tamura

When the scope reaches the hepatic flexure, you will be able to see a bluish spot beyond the intestinal wall. That is the liver. From here, suction air, push the scope, hook the bend with the distal end, and rotate it clockwise to enter the ascending colon (**Fig. 9-2-1**).

If the distal end cannot reach the bend, remove the warp, push the scope while preventing sagging of the transverse colon by applying gentle extra-abdominal pressure of an assistant's hand on the areas above and below the umbilicus, and enter the ascending colon as described above.

125

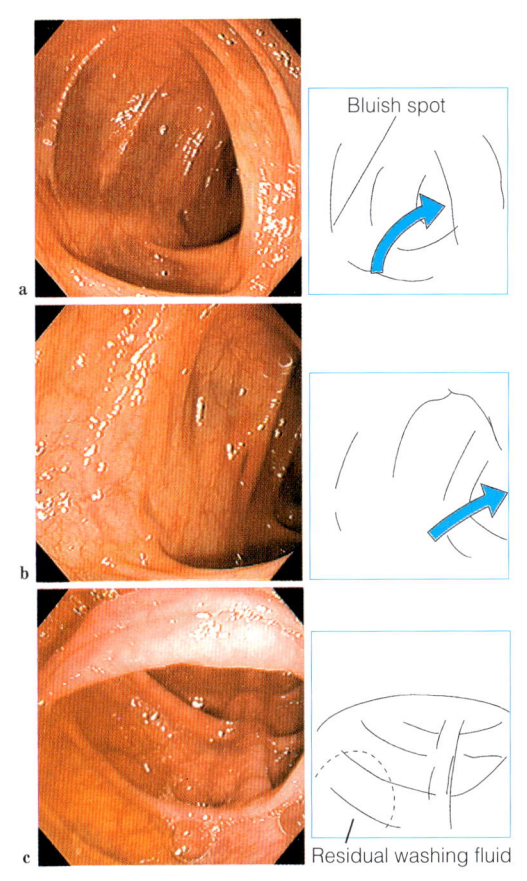

Fig. 9-2-1   Passing through the hepatic flexure
a) Check the direction for entering the bend and advance the scope's distal end toward it.
b) Hook the bend and pass it.
c) The scope enters the ascending colon by passing through the hepatic flexure. Here, residual washing fluid is often observed.

③ Hook the flexure with the scope's distal end

Osamu Tsuruta, Hiroshi Kawano

The most effective technique used to pass through the hepatic flexure is to bring the scope's distal end close enough to the flexure to hook it. Once the flexure is hooked, the scope can be advanced into the ascending colon relatively easily by means of angulation, air suctioning and gentle pushing.

Here, we will describe how to approach, hook and pass the hepatic flexure. Generally, we keep the patient in the supine position in these operations.

1. How to approach and pass through the hepatic flexure by pulling and twisting the scope

After passing the transverse colon bend closest to the hepatic flexure, twist the scope counterclockwise and pull it, while angulating it to get a view of the lumen. In general, this maneuver moves the distal end closer to the hepatic flexure. Now you can use the following techniques to pass through the scope.

1) Passing through the hepatic flexure by twisting the scope clockwise

If the hepatic flexure is already hooked at the time the scope is pulled back, twist the scope clockwise and suction air while keeping the lumen in view to enter the ascending colon. If the hepatic flexure is not already hooked, then you will be unlikely to be able to advance the scope by pushing it. Instead, apply suction or have the patient take a deep breath. This will make it easier to advance the scope and hook the flexure with it.

2) Passing through the hepatic flexure by twisting the scope counterclockwise

If you cannot hook the hepatic flexure using technique 1), twist the scope counterclockwise to view the hepatic flexure in the 12 o'clock direction and suction air. In some cases, this will make it possible to advance the scope's distal end and hook the hepatic flexure with it. In this case, angulating the scope in the 12 o'clock direction often makes it possible to advance the scope in the ascending colon.

3) Hand pressure

If you are not able to hook the hepatic flexure using either technique 1) or

2), applying hand pressure as described below may enable you to hook the hepatic flexure.

  a) Hand pressure to push the right part of the transverse colon up toward the hepatic flexure:

  In this case, refer to the monitor image and press in the direction that the scope's distal end approaches the bend.

  b) Hand pressure to prevent the sigmoid colon from forming a loop:

  In this case, apply pressure to the right lower or central lower abdomen, in the direction toward the pubis.

4) Patient position change

Temporarily putting the patient in the left lateral position and then back in the supine position can help make it easier to perform techniques 1) and 2).

2. How to approach and pass through the hepatic flexure with pushing of the scope

There are cases in which the hepatic flexure cannot be approached even when the scope is pulled back. In these cases, it is necessary to approach the hepatic flexure by pushing the scope using one of the following techniques.

1) Pushing the scope without using hand pressure:

With this technique, simply push the scope to hook the hepatic flexure with it. As this will make the bend in the hepatic flexure more acute, it forces you to sharply angulate the scope without being able to see the lumen in order to advance to the ascending colon. When you reach the ascending colon, pull the scope to straighten out the transverse colon. This technique is accompanied by patient discomfort.

2) Pushing the scope while using hand pressure:

This technique adds hand pressure to technique 1). It is recommended to press the transverse colon up toward the head so that the transverse colon is not sagging while the scope is pushed.

3) Pushing the scope using position change:

Putting the patient in the right lateral position before pushing the scope may make it easier to advance the distal end and hook the hepatic flexure.

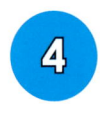

④ Taking advantage of the descending phenomenon of the hepatic flexure, together with hand compression on the abdomen and patient position change

Shinji Tanaka

1. Use of paradoxical movement caused by suction

After passing the scope through the middle part of the transverse colon, you can advance it to the hepatic flexure by keeping it angulated upwards, while suctioning air and pulling back the scope (this is what is called "paradoxical" movement). From there, the scope can be advanced into the ascending colon by suctioning air and having the patient take deep breaths while rotating the scope clockwise.

In doing this, it is also important to let the scope advance naturally by taking advantage of the paradoxical movement caused by the air suctioning. It is important to be careful not to pull too much on the scope's distal end, as this may cause pain to the patient. Instead, let the paradoxical movement move the scope forward.

When the scope is in the proximity of the hepatic flexure, it is important to check the following points:
① Accurately identify the direction in which the scope is to be advanced, based on the three-dimensional anatomy, haustra and innominate grooves on the hepatic flexure.
② Manipulate the scope to move its distal end toward the ascending colon. Provided that there is enough space in the hepatic flexure, the scope can be brought into the ascending colon by rotating it clockwise while continuing to suction air.

2. If you have difficulty entering the ascending colon

If you have difficulty entering the ascending colon:
① First, have the patient take a deep breath. This will cause the hepatic

flexure to descend together with the diaphragm, facilitating insertion of the scope into the ascending colon.

② Apply direct compression (which means using fingers, not the palm, for compression) to **the point where the scope's distal end can be brought closest to the hepatic flexure** (this is the most effective compression point and is usually located slightly to the right of the umbilicus, though this varies depending on the individual). This will prevent the transverse colon from sagging, allowing you to push the scope to insert into the ascending colon.

③ If it is still not possible to enter the ascending colon or if there is not enough space in the hepatic flexure, put the patient in the left lateral position so that the air in the transverse colon collects in the hepatic flexure, then suction the collected air. This often facilitates insertion of the scope into the ascending colon.

④ The right lateral position can also be effective sometimes. This may be because movement of air in the colon helps keep the scope from warping.

As we have seen, the keys to successful insertion include paradoxical movement, taking advantage of the descent of the hepatic flexure following diaphragm contraction from the patient's respiration, and the use of accurate hand compression and patient position changes.

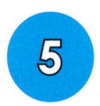

⑤ Using respiratory assistance, patient position change and hand pressure

Eisai Cho

1. Basic maneuver

With a shortened, straightened scope, entrance into the ascending colon from the transverse colon can usually be accomplished by twisting the scope clockwise as if dropping it into the ascending colon.

If you find it difficult to pass through the hepatic flexure, adjust the scope axis so that the minor curve appears at the bottom of the view and the major curve at the top of the view, shorten the scope almost to the near point that the scope is withdrawn, and then twist the scope clockwise to advance it as if dropping it into the ascending colon.

2. Respiratory assistance and patient position change

If insertion is not possible using the basic maneuver described above, use the respiratory assistance technique. Have the patient take a deep breath and hold his or her breath, either in the fully exhaled or fully inhaled status. This may improve the view and facilitate insertion.

If this technique is ineffective, shorten the scope in the transverse colon, adjust the axis, and push in the scope if the distal end can be advanced — even if this results in stretching of the intestinal tract. A similar effect to that obtained with respiratory assistance can sometimes be obtained by changing the patient position to the left lateral position. This position can improve the view of the hepatic flexure and facilitate insertion of the scope.

Using both techniques of respiratory assistance and position change together is also effective (**Fig. 9-5-1**).

3. Hand pressure

If none of the techniques described above proves effective, you can try using hand pressure. First, shorten and straighten the scope near the hepatic flexure. Next, to prevent stretching of the transverse colon, apply hand pressure on the center of the upper abdomen from the front toward the

Fig. 9-5-1
a) Endoscopic image of the hepatic flexure in the left lateral position
b) Endoscopic image of a) when patient has taken a deep breath

upper part of the back so that the transverse colon does not sag (T-point).

If this technique is not appropriate, apply hand pressure to preventing stretching of the sigmoid colon (S-point). After shortening the scope, have the assistant spread both hands and press a wide area in the left lower abdomen from the front toward the back.

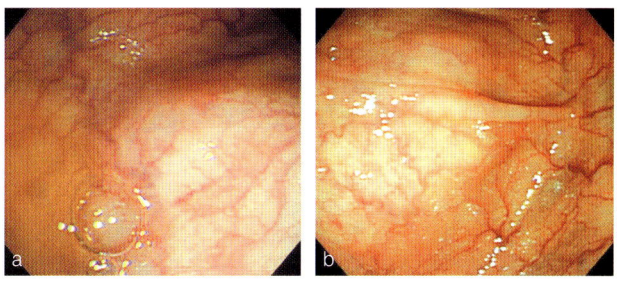

Alternatively, you can apply pressure on both the transverse colon and sigmoid colon simultaneously (T- and S-points).

4. Sliding tube

If all the techniques above are still ineffective, use a sliding tube. Attach a sliding tube to the scope, and slide it along the scope as far as the descending colon after the scope is shortened and straightened from the sigmoid to the descending colon. As this inhibits stretching of the sigmoid colon, the scope can easily be passed through the hepatic flexure.

Scope insertion to the ascending colon can be facilitated by twisting the scope clockwise, by using the respiratory assistance based on deep breath of the patient, by changing the patient position to the left lateral position, by pushing the scope while stretching the intestinal tract, or by applying hand pressure to the transverse colon (T-point).

Occasionally, after finding that all of the methods above are ineffective, you may attempt to push in the scope and discover that the working length of the scope is insufficient, though this is very rare. If this happens, attach a long sliding tube to a long scope and insert it.

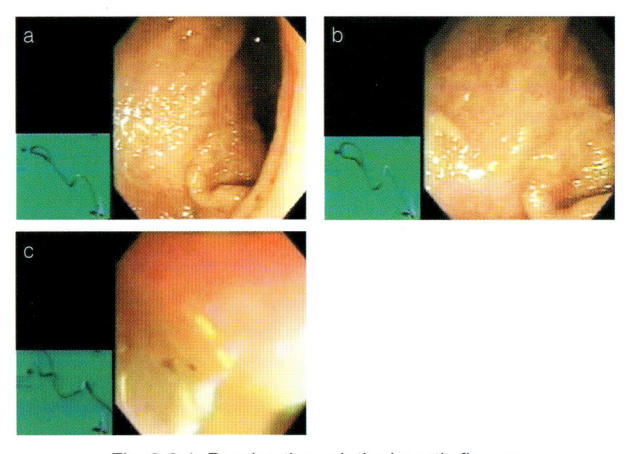

⑥ Key tips on passing through the hepatic flexure

Yusuke Saitoh

Key tips
- Have the assistant observe the image on the monitor to find the point where the scope approaches closest to the hepatic flexure. Pass through the hepatic flexure while the assistant presses that point.
- Also use deep breathing and patient position change.

Normally, all you need to do to pass through the hepatic flexure is suction

Fig. 9-6-1 Passing through the hepatic flexure
a) Sufficient suction and pullback brings the scope to the hepatic flexure. The ascending colon is visible on the right.
b) When the hepatic flexure cannot be passed through because one fold still needs to be crossed, have the assistant find the pressure point where the wall comes closest to the scope and pass the fold while the assistant applies hand pressure. Having the patient take a deep breath or change their position can also be helpful.
c) Hand pressure brings the wall close to the scope. Rotating the scope clockwise advances it into the ascending colon.

enough air and pull back the scope. The ascending colon can usually be reached by clockwise rotation of the scope (**Fig. 9-6-1a**). If the hepatic flexure of the patient is located at a high position (which occurs more frequently with elderly patients), insertion may not be possible, leaving only one fold to be crossed.

In such a case, have the assistant observe the monitor image to find the point where the scope most closely approaches the hepatic flexure (this point is often in the right hypochondrium, but sometimes hand pressure on a point between the epigastric region and the left hypochondrium is more effective), and pass through the hepatic flexure while the assistant applies hand pressure to that point (pressing gently with a single finger should be sufficient) (**Fig. 9-6-1b, c**). Having the patient take a deep breath or change their posture can also be helpful.

It is usually not difficult to pass through the ascending colon and reach the cecum, but insertion may be difficult if the patient is obese and the sigmoid colon and/or transverse colon is sagging. In such a case, compression on the area around the umbilicus may prevent loop formation in the sigmoid colon and transverse colon, facilitating insertion into the cecum. Deep breathing and position change are also useful.

10. From the Cecum to the Terminal Ileum

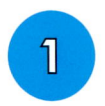

1 Indication for terminal ileum insertion and insertion frequency

Yuji Inoue

1. Before insertion into the terminal ileum (insertion from ascending colon to cecum)

After inserting the scope into the ascending colon, pull back the scope slightly, suction some air in the intestinal tract and push the transverse colon upward. This makes it possible for you to insert the scope all the way to cecum in one go. Provided that no loop forms, you should always be able to observe the ileocecal valve on the left side of the monitor image.

Sometimes, in videos of colonoscopic insertion presented at society meetings, the ileocecal valve is shown on the right side of the screen; this simply indicates that a loop has formed somewhere in the colon. Considering that in 99% of cases the loop can be removed in the process of insertion to the ascending colon, such a video actually presents a failed case.

Before starting insertion into the terminal ileum, it is important to be sure that there is no loop. The probability that there is no loop is high when: ① the scope maintains torque trackability; ② the ileocecal valve can be observed on the left; ③ the scope length from the anal verge is about 70 cm.

2. Insertion into the terminal ileum

Terminal ileum insertion is indicated for diseases frequently found in the ileocecal region such as Crohn's disease and Behcet's disease, as well as for close examination of the source of melena.

Some of the contributors to this book may argue that insertion into the terminal ileum is critical. In my experience, however, when one excludes cases where terminal ileum insertion is indicated, less than 50% of cases require insertion into the terminal ileum. This is because 70% of the cases I examine are repeaters and that the rate of detection of disease in the terminal ileum observation is actually low.

As I do not use anesthesia in examinations and the monitor is placed in front of the patient, I am happy to explain to them what they are seeing on the screen should they wish to observe. About half the patients are interested in monitoring what's on the screen. Before insertion into the terminal ileum, I explain to them that this lip-like organ is the valve between the small and large intestines, and the organ beyond it is the small intestine.

Normally, with patients who do not wish to monitor the procedure, I omit scope insertion into the terminal ileum. However, mastery of the terminal ileum insertion technique is essential for a colonoscopist, so we always ask beginners and intermediate colonoscopists at our center to insert the scope to the terminal ileum.

There is a trick to insertion into the terminal ileum. As it is located at the side of the ascending colon, you are not likely to be able to insert the scope simply by pushing the scope; all this does is cause pain to the patient. Typically, the ileocecal valve has a lip-like or papilla-like shape. When it has a papilla-like shape, the valve is closed, so blindly pushing the scope results in nothing but excessive stretching of the colon.

Instead, the scope should be applied gently to the valve, as if placing the scope on the valve. Insufflate a small amount of air at this point opens the ileocecal valve and the scope enters a little into the valve as if being absorbed.

Now, you can insert the scope into the terminal ileum by pushing the scope very gently. The actually observable length of the ileum varies greatly between individuals, extending from about 10 cm to about 50 cm (I was once able to diagnose Meckel's diverticulum with a colonoscope).

2 Conditions required for scope insertion into terminal ileum

Sumio Tsuda

For smooth insertion of the scope into the terminal ileum, the bending section on the scope's distal end should have reached the cecum located on the oral side of Bauhin's valve as shown in **Fig. 10-2-1**. If the bending section on the scope's distal end cannot reach inside the cecum on the oral side of Bauhin's valve (**Fig. 10-2-2**), insertion into the terminal ileum will not be possible. To achieve this, insert the scope by shortening the extent from the rectum to the ascending colon.

1. Scope insertion into the terminal ileum

Once the scope has reached the cecum, angulate it so that the distal end points towards Bauhin's valve, which will be visible on the left side of the monitor image, and move it forward. This usually makes it possible to easily insert the scope into the terminal ileum. Bauhin's valve may be visible on the right, top or bottom of the monitor image depending on the scope insertion angle. Insertion into the terminal ileum is also possible in these cases by angulating the scope accordingly.

However, if the scope shaft is deviated outside (**Fig. 10-2-3** ①) or the scope is too flexible and retroflexed inside the cecum (**Fig. 10-2-3** ②), insertion into the terminal ileum may not be possible. If this is the case, changing the patient position to the left lateral position will usually make it possible to advance the scope. The prone position and/or hand pressure may also be effective.

2. Scope insertion inside the ileum

After the scope's distal end has crossed Bauhin's valve and entered the terminal ileum, advance the scope slowly, while monitoring the lumen in the center of the screen. The bends can be passed by suctioning air and angulating the scope. Do not push the scope forcibly. In general, the scope insertion method inside the ileum is more or less the same as inside the colon.

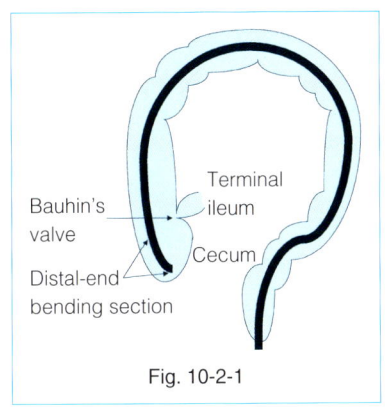

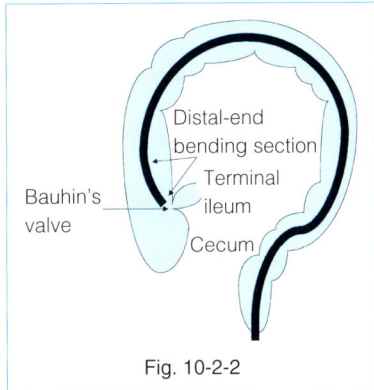

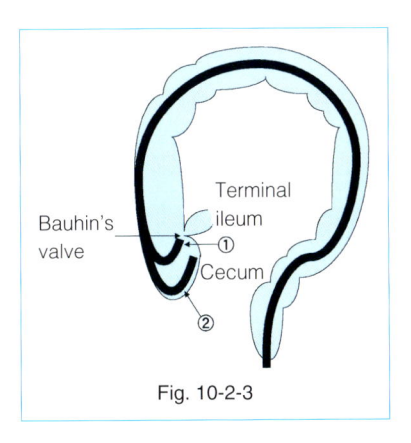

Fig. 10-2-1

Fig. 10-2-2

Fig. 10-2-3

③ Scope insertion from the cecum to the ileum

Osamu Tsuruta, Hiroshi Kawano

1. Straighten the scope

Insertion of the scope into the terminal ileum by passing through the ileocecal valve is a procedure that requires a combination of careful maneuvers, including delicate rotation and angulation. In order to execute these maneuvers successfully, it is critical to make sure the scope is straight so that the movements of your hand are transmitted directly to the scope's distal end.

2. Insert the scope's distal end to the bottom of the cecum

3. Pull the scope so its distal end slides across the lower lip of the ileocecal valve (Fig. 10-3-1)

From the bottom of the cecum, pull the scope so that its distal end slides along the lower lip of the ileocecal valve. It is recommended to twist the scope counterclockwise during pullback.

4. Confirm the ileocecal orifice (Fig. 10-3-2)

5. Confirm the entrance of the terminal ileum (Fig. 10-3-3)

Continue rotating the scope counterclockwise and pull it. The entrance of the terminal ileum will come into view.

6. Insert the scope into the terminal ileum (Fig. 10-3-4)

While observing the entrance of the terminal ileum on the monitor, push the scope into the terminal ileum.

7. Insert the scope further toward the oral side of the ileum (Fig. 10-3-5)

To pass the bend in the ileum, insert the scope's distal end slightly beyond the bend, angulate the distal end toward the bend and pull back the scope. The scope will advance toward the oral side.

Normally, a colonoscope can only be inserted about 15 to 20 cm from the entrance of the terminal ileum, but the operation above makes possible insertion into the ileum in most cases.

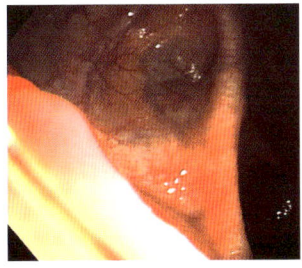

Fig. 10-3-1 Pulling the scope so that as if the distal end slides along the lower lip of the ileocecal valve

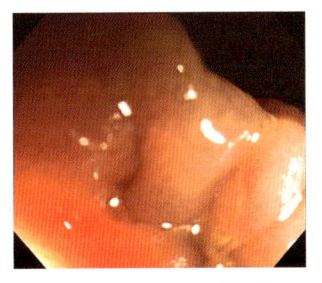

Fig. 10-3-2 Entrance of the ileum

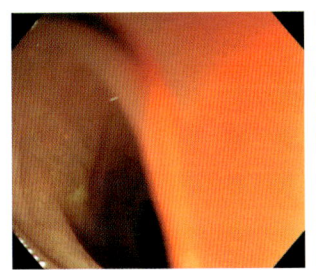

Fig. 10-3-3 Entrance of the terminal ileum

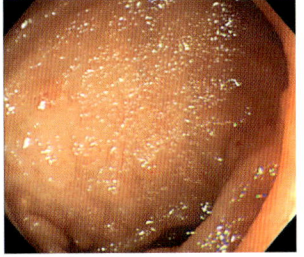

Fig. 10-3-4 Terminal ileum

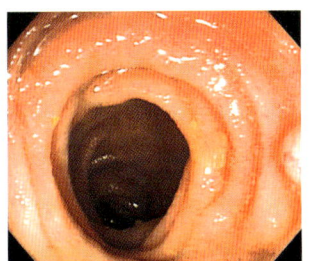

Fig. 10-3-5 Terminal ileum beyond the bend

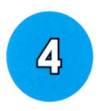

④ Appendix orifice, the terminal point of colonoscopy

Satoru Tamura

Insertion from the ascending colon to the cecum is usually easy. However, if spasms are severe or if the sigmoid colon and/or transverse colon sags too easily, you may need to apply gentle extra-abdominal pressure of an assistant's hand and/or ask the patient to breathe deeply.

The terminal point of colonoscopy is the cecum, so looking down Bauhin's valve from the ascending colon should not be considered the final stage in observation. In order to avoid the possibility of overlooking cecal lesions, it is important to observe the appendix orifice. Inserting the scope from Bauhin's valve to the terminal ileum is easy when you can look down the aperture of the valve; however, if it the aperture is hidden by the upper lip, you will have to proceed blindly to some extent.

Once you have inserted the scope to the cecum, insert the scope into the terminal ileum by angulating it upward, pulling it toward Bauhin's valve and correcting the angulation immediately before the upper lip comes into view (**Fig. 10-4-1**). After entering the terminal ileum, the villi of the small intestine can be observed by means of dye spraying.

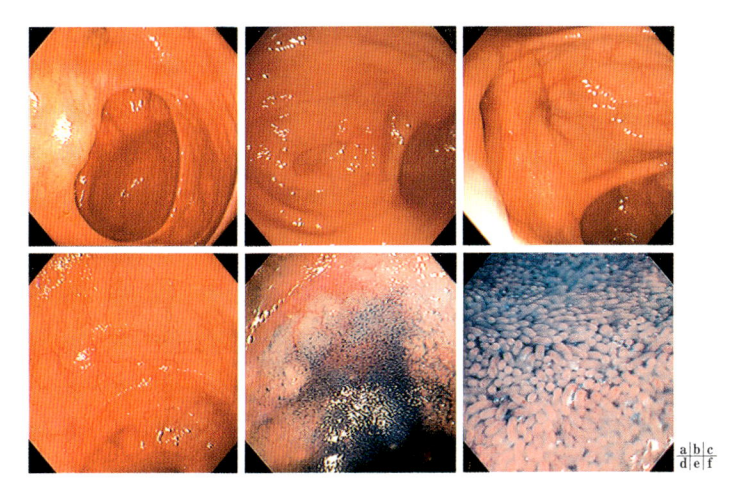

Fig. 10-4-1 Cecum, Bauhin's valve and terminal ileum
a) Bauhin's valve, looked down from the ascending colon
b) Appendix orifice
c) Bauhin's valve: Correct the angulation immediately before the upper lip comes into view, and then insert the scope into the terminal ileum.
d) Terminal ileum
e) Dye-sprayed image of terminal ileum
f) Villi of the terminal ileum after dye spraying. Magnifying observation image obtained with a magnifying videoscope (Olympus CF-200Z)

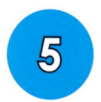

⑤ Important tips in the path from cecum to terminal ileum

Yusuke Saitoh

Important tips
- If the scope reaches the cecum without forming a loop, the ileocecal valve can usually be seen in the 8 to 9 o'clock direction.
- Suction excess air from the cecum.
- After passing the ileocecal valve, pull back the scope gradually, while rotating it counterclockwise, and hook the upper lip with the scope. Alternatively, slide the scope along the lower lip of the ileocecal valve and angulate the scope upward to insert it into the terminal ileum.

If the scope has reached the cecum without twisting or looping, in the shape of the number "7", then ileocecal valve can usually be observed in the 8 to 9 o'clock direction (**Fig. 10-5-1a**).
The tips for insertion into the terminal ileum are as follows:
- Suction excess air from the cecum.
- Insert the scope until it passes through the ileocecal valve.
- Pull back the scope gradually, while rotating it counterclockwise, and hook the upper lip of the ileocecal valve with the scope. Alternatively, slide the scope along the lower lip of the ileocecal valve and angulate the scope upward to insert it into the terminal ileum.

Usually a close-up image is displayed on the monitor during passage of the ileocecal valve until the point where the scope enters the terminal ileum (**Fig. 10-5-1b**). After a series of close-up images have slid by, pull back the scope slightly, insufflate air and confirm that the scope is inserted in the terminal ileum (**Fig. 10-5-1c**).

If the patient has recently had a laparotomy or has an inflammatory bowel disease such as Crohn's disease, insertion into the ileum may be difficult because adhesion makes the angle formed between the ileocecal

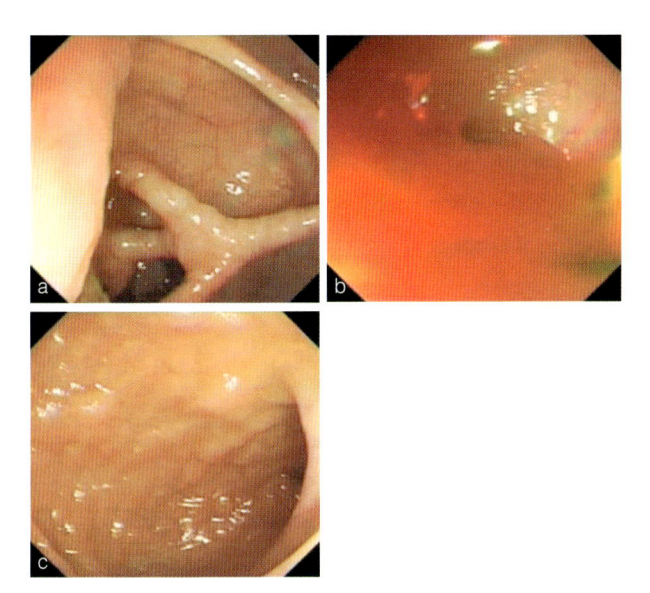

Fig. 10-5-1 From cecum to terminal ileum
a) If the scope reaches the cecum without forming a loop, the ileocecal valve can usually be observed in the 8 to 9 o'clock direction.
b) After passing the ileocecal valve, pull back the scope gradually, while rotating it counterclockwise, and hook the upper lip with the scope. Alternatively, slide the scope along the lower lip of the ileocecal valve and angulate the scope upward to insert it pass through the ileocecal valve.
c) The scope reaches the terminal ileum where the lymphatic system is highly developed and small-intestinal villi are present.

valve and terminal ileum more acute. In this case, apply hand pressure by finding the point in the ascending colon or ileocecal region where you can see the ileocecal valve in close-up on the monitor and where pushing the scope can transmit the force to the distal end. This may enable insertion into the ileum.

However, insertion into the deep part of the ileum is usually difficult because the small intestine is not fixed. Balloon enteroscopy is recommended for the deep insertion of the ileum.

⑥ Getting from the cecum to the terminal ileum by preserving the scope's freedom of movement

Shinji Tanaka

1. Straightening the scope is essential

In order to successfully insert the scope from the cecum to the terminal ileum, the scope must be straightened beforehand and kept straight throughout. If a loop forms, insertion into the terminal ileum will be painful for the patient.

To insert the scope into the terminal ileum, first suction as much air as possible air from the region around the cecum and ascending colon to maintain the scope's freedom of movement. Suctioning air from the cecum also helps facilitates direct view of the ileocecal valve orifice.

In this condition, the scope can be inserted into the ileocecal valve orifice by angling the scope's distal end toward the mesentery. As the thickness of the ileocecal valve can vary significantly — from very thick to so thin that identification from the haustra is extremely difficult, make sure that you have identified the valve before insertion.

2. Tips for insertion into the ileocecal valve orifice

In some cases, insertion of the scope's distal end into the ileocecal valve orifice may fail because the scope bends. If this happens, hand compression on the lower abdomen can be effective. Changing the patient position to the supine or left (or right) lateral position can also be helpful as this moves the air inside the intestines, making insertion into the terminal ileum easier.

11. How to Deal with Cases Where Insertion Is Difficult
1) Postoperative Adhesion

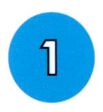

① Never use force to manipulate the scope

Yasumoto Suzuki

1. Regions where postoperative adhesion occurs frequently

Postoperative adhesions in the sigmoid colon and transverse colon tend to make scope insertion more difficult. Both of these organs have mesenteries that make them highly mobile. However, once an adhesion is produced, the intestinal tract will be set in a stretched, bent or twisted state, making insertion difficult. Nevertheless, it is unusual for total colonoscopy to be rendered completely impossible due to adhesion, except in very severe cases. In other words, there is no reason to give up without trying.

2. Postoperative adhesions in the sigmoid colon

The sigmoid colon includes two major bends — the S-top and the SD junction. These two positions are usually the critical points in insertion into the sigmoid colon, but if the patient has postoperative adhesions, additional bends may be produced that are difficult to pass. In such cases, trying to continue insertion simply by pushing not only makes it impossible to advance the scope any further, but also makes it impossible to shorten the stretched intestinal tract.

What is required here is a method of insertion that does not reduce the force transmitted to the distal end of the scope. In general, there is less attenuation of force transmitted to the scope's distal end in the sigmoid colon, but this does not apply to postoperative adhesion cases.

Sometimes, almost all of the force transmitted to the distal end is lost the moment the scope enters the sigmoid colon. In such cases, do not attempt to insert the scope all the way at once. It is more effective to focus on transmitting force to the scope's distal end, inserting it a little at a time by gently pushing and pulling repeatedly. This technique requires a great deal of patience, but it is important to maintain your concentration. Just remember that you will reach the splenic flexure eventually.

3. Postoperative adhesions in the transverse colon

Normally, the key to passage of the transverse colon is the bend in the center. Usually, this bend is utilized as a fulcrum in which the transverse colon is straightened by lifting the middle section and passing the hepatic flexure.

Unfortunately, it is not quite so easy with postoperative adhesion cases. Because postoperative adhesion makes it impossible to lift the center of the transverse colon, the most effective method is to push the scope through the center of the transverse colon and the hepatic flexure and then lift the transverse colon by utilizing the hepatic flexure as the fulcrum.

If it becomes impossible to advance the scope in the middle due to a decrease in the transmission of force to the scope's distal end, use hand pressure or a sliding tube to prevent the sigmoid colon from stretching. This often makes it possible to pass through the hepatic flexure.

4. Cautions for postoperative adhesion cases

If strong resistance is felt during scope insertion in a case with postoperative adhesion, be careful not to use force to try and insert the scope because this is one of the most frequent causes of perforation. It is not necessary to give up the procedure, but unnecessary risks must always be avoided.

2 Carefully pass each fold, using as little air as possible

Norihiro Hamamoto

1. Use a slim scope for post-gynecological cancer removal or post-C-section cases

The postoperative cases that pose the most difficulty are those in which the patients have been left with intrapelvic bowel adhesions after gynecological cancer removal or C-section because the sigmoid colon is adhered to itself or to the small intestine.

Typically, the bend between the S-top and sigmoid colon is very acute and complex. When a severe adhesion is anticipated, the patient should be given a sedative, as well as an antispasmodic, before beginning the procedure.

The insertion method itself is the same as in ordinary cases, but it is important to point out that, in the approach to the descending colon, inserting the scope slowly and carefully will ultimately facilitate pain-free insertion in a short period of time.

As a rule, you should never insert the scope by force. Using as little air as possible, repeat the angulation maneuver frequently and insert the scope, while keeping it straight, by folding the intestinal tract. In cases of advanced adhesion, the lumen is narrower and scope operability is extremely poor. All you can do in such a case is to carefully pass each fold in the lumen by making use of downward angulations.

Until the scope enters the descending colon, hook every fold in every bend with the scope and insert the scope carefully with precise angulation maneuvers in the up, down, left and right directions. When resistance or deflection is encountered, try to straighten it carefully so that the scope does not withdraw.

It is important to be patient as you repeat this series of maneuvers. A slim scope is effective both for passing through an acute bend and reducing patient pain if a loop forms. As a narrower-diameter scope is more likely to form a loop than scopes with wider diameters, hand pressure should be applied in the public symphysis region. Hand pressure is also effective with slender women. Even when shortening and straightening in the segment from the S-top to the distal sigmoid is not possible, try to keep the loop as small as possible if one forms. Again, in this case, the amount of air should be kept to a minimum.

2. Post-colectomy cases

After rectal or sigmoid cancer surgery, the intestinal tract is linear so scope insertion is even easier than in ordinary cases. Simply twisting the scope slightly clockwise is usually enough to get the scope to the descending colon. With patients undergoing colectomy of the transverse colon or right-side colon, adhesions inside the pelvic cavity are usually quite minor so the chances of a difficult insertion are relatively low.

3. Post-gastrectomy or post-cholecystectomy cases

With these cases, the transverse colon is stuck to the abdominal wall. Although this is not usually a problem for insertion up to the transverse colon, shortening is sometimes difficult in the segment from the middle of the transverse colon to the hepatic flexure, in which case you may have to push the scope. As long as the patient does not complain about pain, you can continue pushing but make sure to reduce the amount of air as much as possible.

In all of the procedures above, the risk of perforation should be considered high if strong resistance is felt or if the patient complains about pain. In such cases, you will have to discontinue the examination.

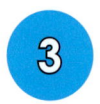

③ Always assume that an adhesion may be present before insertion

Hiroshi Kashida

Patients who have had an appendectomy (particularly a case complicated with peritonitis) or gynecological surgery sometimes have adhesions in the Rs-S junction and/or sigmoid colon, which can interfere with insertion of the colonoscope. Patients who have undergone gastrectomy or cholecystectomy often have adhesions in the transverse colon.

Unfortunately, there is usually no way to know whether an adhesion is present or not before examination, nor is there any special insertion technique to deal with adhesion. The presence of an adhesion is usually indicated by an extremely acute bend in the intestinal tract and difficulty in moving the intestinal tract when attempting to shorten it.

If you stick to the basics when performing insertion, you should be able to complete an examination successfully without noticing the presence of an adhesion even when one is present.

1. Air suction and repeated shortening little by little are important

As the intestinal tract is fixed at many points if adhesions are present, it is virtually impossible and very risky to try to fold a long length of tract all at once or to perfectly straighten the tract. The more air is insufflated, the more acute the bends become since the intestinal tract is constricted at the fixed points like a chain of sausages. In such a case, it is necessary to minimize the amount of air and attenuate the bends at the fixed points by repeatedly shortening the tract a little at a time.

2. Is hand pressure useful?

When the intestinal tract is fixed, it is hard to move it with hand pressure and strong pressure may cause pain. However, hand pressure can be effective in regions without adhesion.

3. Is patient posture change useful?

Since the intestinal tract is hard to fold and hand pressure is not really reliable, patient posture change is often the best way to facilitate insertion. Changing the posture can attenuate the degree of bending of the fixed points and move excessive air in the intestinal tract. However, there are cases in which a position change in a direction opposite from usual is more effective depending on the number and locations of the fixed points. You will have to find the best posture for each fixed points through trial and error.

4. What kind of scope should be used?

A slim, flexible scope is sometimes more suitable for passage through a region with adhesions. However, once this region has been passed, subsequent insertion is usually easier with a stiffer scope.

5. There is no quick solution for adhesion cases

Since the location of adhesions and the number of fixed points vary from one case to the next, there is no one technique that can be applicable to every case. You will have to put all your knowledge and skill to the task in each case in order to perform a successful intubation. There is always a chance that you will have to deal with a case with adhesions. The most important is to assume that any case may include adhesions and always stick to the basics of insertion in your daily practice.

6. Do not blame everything on adhesions

When the scope cannot be inserted as expected or if the patient complains of pain, many endoscopists tend to blame it on poor preparation, an excessively long intestine, or adhesions. Try to avoid thinking this way. You should always be prepared to admit that your skills may be insufficient. On the other hand, if the presence of an adhesion is strongly suspected and there is abnormal resistance to insertion, do not try to push too hard and be willing to give up the procedure to avoid the risk of injuring the patient.

4 Areas where insertion is difficult vary depending on whether and where the patient has undergone surgery

Masahiro Igarashi

1. After gynecological surgery

Adhesions in the sigmoid colon are common in patients who have undergone gynecological surgery, making insertion difficult in the segment from the sigmoid colon to the descending colon. In such cases, the safest thing to do is to use a slim scope right from the outset.

As pain is also to be expected, preprocedural administration of a sedative or analgesic should also be considered. I usually obtain intravenous access and administer about 3-4 mg of Dormicum®. The reason for using a slim scope is that its distal end is highly mobile and easy to go through the colon even in the presence of an adhesion.

Furthermore, even if a loop forms, the scope's flexibility can prevent the intestinal tract from stretching excessively and reduce the potential for exfoliation of adhesions. In fact, insertion that would be difficult for an ordinary scope can often be made possible simply by switching to a slim scope.

2. After gastrectomy

Difficulties in passage occur often in the extent from the splenic flexure to the transverse colon. Even after passing the hepatic flexure, the scope's distal end may not be able to reach the cecum in some cases. As the transverse colon of a post-gastrectomy patient is often fixed, it can be difficult to advance the distal end and a loop could easily form in the transverse colon as shown in **Fig. 11-1-4-1**.

Nevertheless, even when a loop forms, it is important to repeat the maneuver of pulling and straightening the scope after passing through a bend. If a loop does form, hand pressure can help prevent the loop from

| Adhesion in the splenic flexure | Adhesion in the transverse colon | Adhesion in the hepatic flexure |

Fig. 11-1-4-1 Pattern of insertion difficulty in the transverse colon after gastrectomy

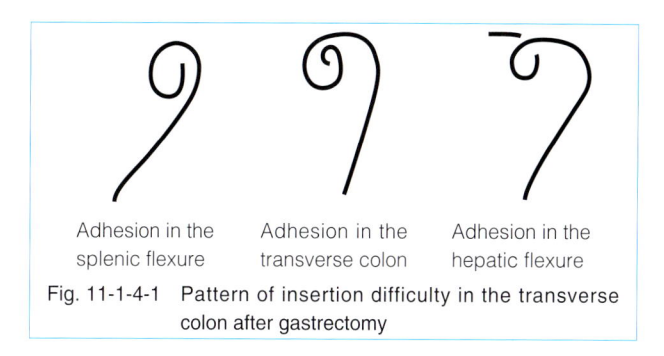

extending, as well as transmitting propulsive force to the distal end.

3. After cholecystectomy

In this case, problems can occur in the hepatic flexure. Adhesions in the hepatic flexure often make it difficult to successfully negotiate passage using conventional techniques. When hand pressure on the right hypochondrium is used, the scope's distal end will normally slide smoothly through the hepatic flexure.

Unfortunately, this is often ineffective if the patient has undergone cholecystectomy. The best solution in this case is to use the push method as shown in **Fig. 11-1-4-2**. In case hand pressure on the right hypochondrium is effective, the scope tip will slide smoothly through the hepatic flexure.

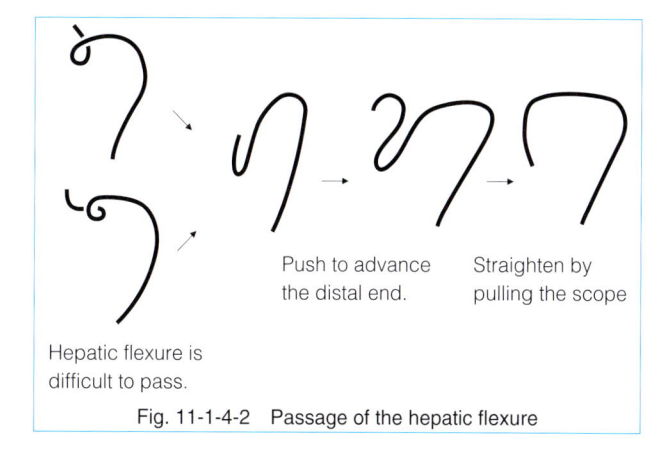

Hepatic flexure is difficult to pass.

Push to advance the distal end.

Straighten by pulling the scope

Fig. 11-1-4-2 Passage of the hepatic flexure

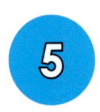

⑤ Tips for insertion in postoperative adhesion cases

Yusuke Saitoh

Important tips
- Before starting colonoscopy (or on receiving an examination order), confirm the detailed procedures and the potential for adhesion by checking the patient's history for peritonitis, gynecological diseases, etc.
- Never take any risks with adhesion cases. Be prepared to end the examination before completion.
- Use conscious sedation.
- Use a malleable or Variable Stiffness scope with a small diameter of about 10 mm or less.

Typically, those cases that pose the most difficulty in insertion involve postoperative adhesions. Before starting colonoscopy (or on receiving an examination order), confirm the detailed procedures and the potential for adhesion by checking the patient's history for peritonitis, gynecological diseases, etc. If the patient has previously undergone a colonoscopy, review the results.

Typical observations that may indicate the presence of adhesions:
① The patient complains of abnormal pain during normal insertion operation.
② When a loop has formed in the sigmoid colon, the patient complains of pain during attempt to release the loop (which usually consists of pullback with clockwise rotation).
③ A loop in the sigmoid colon cannot be removed.
④ The paradoxical movement cannot always be achieved in the right part of the transverse colon even when no reverse loop is formed (pulling back the scope cannot bring it to the hepatic flexure).
⑤ Insertion from the ascending colon to the cecum is difficult.

⑥ Insertion from the cecum to the terminal ileum is difficult.

Any of these observations can indicate an adhesion. When an adhesion is suspected, the important thing is to avoid the risk. If you sedate a patient who has adhesions in order to perform forcible total colonoscopy, it may lead to complications including mucosal rupture, bleeding, perforation and intraperitoneal bleeding due to mechanical exfoliation of adhesion.

Rather than subject the patient to severe pain and potential complications, it is better to abandon the colonoscopy and order an alternative examination such as a barium enema fluoroscopy or CT colography. It is also important to be willing to request a specialist to perform the examination.

However, when a colonoscopic examination is absolutely necessary, I recommend using either or both of the following methods:

① Apply conscious sedation (such as midazolam) before the patient complains about strong pain.

② Use a thin scope with a diameter of about 10 mm (Olympus PCF-PQ260L/I or PCF-PH190L/I) or a Variable Stiffness scope (Olympus PCF-Q260AZI or PCF-Q180AL/I, PCF-H180AL/I, PCF-H190L/I).

In some cases, even when one of these scope models is used together with sedation, it may still not be possible to reach the cecum. Again, it is important to remember that you should never run the risk.

6 Take a surgical history in the pre-procedure interview

Satoru Tamura

Adhesions occur either as a postoperative phenomenon or as a result of advanced cancer. With patients who have undergone ordinary gynecological operations, it is rare that postoperative adhesions make insertion into the sigmoid colon impossible. However, among patients who have suffered severe peritonitis or undergone gynecological surgery accompanied by a wide range of pelvic cavity manipulations, there are cases in which unnatural and acute bends hinder intestinal shortening and observation is only possible as far as the sigmoid colon.

Among patients who have undergone upper abdominal (gastric or biliary) surgery, there are cases in which an adhesion in the transverse colon forms an unnatural bend and makes it impossible to insert the scope past that region. This happens most frequently in the middle of the transverse colon. It is very difficult to advance past such a bend using the push technique, and attempting to do so can cause considerable pain.

To get through such a bend, you must use the shortening technique to approach the bend and then hook the fold on the adhesion with the scope's distal end. Sometimes it is a good idea to attach a transparent hood to the distal end.

In any case, you should always take the surgical history of each patient in the pre-procedure interview to identify any situations that may arise. If it looks like colonoscopy will be impossible or too risky, abandon the procedure and observe the right side of the colon using barium enema.

Some advanced cancers may infiltrate in the serosal side and adhere with the intestinal tract on the anal side, forming a very acute, hairpin-curved bend. Be careful with such cases, as well.

11. How to Deal with Cases Where Insertion Is Difficult
2) Dolichocolon (Sigmoid Colon, Transverse Colon)

1 Dolichocolon and air insufflation

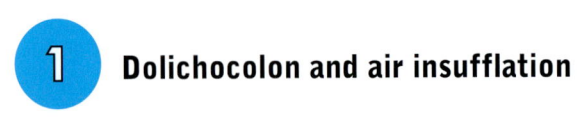

Hiroyuki Tsukagoshi

Generally, you can use the same insertion methods for cases with dolichocolon as for other cases (except cases with advanced adhesions and extreme obesity). Dolichocolon does not always mean that insertion is difficult. If you know that a patient has a long colon, you can deal with it by insufflating less air than usual.

1. Misunderstanding on hooking the fold

The correct hooking-the-fold technique involves finding the lumen by pulling the scope while insufflating a small amount of air. Many beginners, however, insufflate too much air when attempting to straighten the scope. This stretches the sigmoid colon and results in the formation of a hairpin curve in the middle of the sigmoid colon. Once the sigmoid colon has been stretched to the limit, it is very difficult to shorten it. It is important to minimize the amount of air when you start this technique.

2. If the colon is stretched to the limit

Once the colon has been stretched all the way, shortening is difficult. The only thing you can do at this point is to push the scope to the SD junction. Using patient position change and hand pressure, slowly advance the scope a little at a time by releasing the angulation knob in the neutral direction from the fully upward-angulated status.

Once the scope reaches the SD junction, you can start trying to shorten the colon. Endoscopists with more advanced skills may be able to bring the descending colon into view by pulling the scope at a point before the SD junction; however, if the angle and direction are not correct, this simply results in withdrawal of the scope.

Pushing the scope in any part of the intestinal tract will result in the formation of a hairpin curve. When a beginner tries to pull the scope, the scope often comes right out due to the excessive amount of air in the tract. If scope pulling fails after a few attempts, switch to the push technique. In this case, push the scope by angulating it upward until the descending colon comes in the view.

When the descending colon is visible, perform right-turn shortening while suctioning enough air to facilitate the maneuver. However, as this technique is accompanied by a risk of perforation, it is important to master the correct method as quickly as you can.

3. Transverse colon

Insertion in the transverse colon is not difficult, if insertion into the splenic flexure has been performed correctly. Incorrect insertion into the splenic flexure can result in the formation of a loop that hinders subsequent movement through the transverse colon.

Air is less of a problem in the transverse colon, even if there is a fair amount of it. Rotate the scope counterclockwise in the middle of the transverse colon to view the entrance into the right side of the colon from the 12 o'clock direction. Alternate between suction and shortening.

Entrance into the ascending colon from the hepatic flexure is easy if the scope's distal end can contact the wall that is farthest away when the right side of the colon is shortened. If the wall cannot be contacted, immediately start pushing the scope. Push down the transverse colon until you reach the pelvic cavity, then hook the ascending colon with the scope's distal end and shorten the transverse colon. It is important not to spend too much time trying to straighten the scope.

② Measures to be taken before and after sigmoid colon insertion

Sumio Tsuda

1. What is dolichocolon?

There is no established definition of dolichocolon as far as colonoscopy is concerned. This section explains what to do when the sigmoid colon is long and has complex contours as shown in **Fig. 11-2-2-1**, making insertion impossible using the shortening technique alone.

2. Steps to take before insertion into the sigmoid colon

If an N-loop has formed but you are able to advance the scope's distal end into the descending colon and splenic flexure using the push operation, then there is nothing to worry about. Similarly, when the scope forms an α-loop, there is nothing to worry about if you can decrease the loop by means of hand pressure and optimum scope manipulation and advance the scope into the descending colon and splenic flexure.

This does not mean that insertion can always be performed successfully when an α-loop is formed. Quite often, this is not the case. When an α-loop cannot be formed, insertion is made difficult when the scope cannot be advanced due to a loop formed by the push operation. In such a case, applying the right amount of hand pressure in the right position can make a big difference. The compression point is usually around the center of the line connecting the anterior superior iliac spine and the umbilicus. In any case, find the point where the scope can be advanced with gentle pressure (enough pressure to cause the intestinal tract on the monitor image to come closer) and compress it with a relatively strong force to advance the scope.

If a bend is encountered, hook it with the scope's distal end and decrease the loop by means of scope shaft rotation and pullback operation. Repeat these scope manipulations to advance the distal end

2) Dolichocolon (Sigmoid Colon, Transverse Colon) *163*

through the descending colon to the splenic flexure.

Needless to say, it is important to avoid causing pain to the patient and to avoid excessive insufflation. Manipulate the scope in sync with the patient's breathing and use lubricant to make the scope slide more easily. It is recommended that you use a scope with a soft tube for push operations, as it is much safer and less painful.

3. Steps to take after sigmoid colon insertion

To insert the scope into the deep part of the colon after passing through the sigmoid colon, you have to straighten the sigmoid colon with the scope as shown in **Fig. 11-2-2-2** and keep it straight.

This is not easy without some experience in the case of dolichosigmoid. It is also important to take advantage of fluoroscopy and the endoscope position detection system. In the case of dolichosigmoid, it can even be hard to keep the scope straight. Deep insertion in such a case may be assisted by hand pressure and patient position change, but it can also be helpful to use a sliding tube or a Variable Stiffness scope, which allows you to adjust the flexibility of the scope's insertion tube.

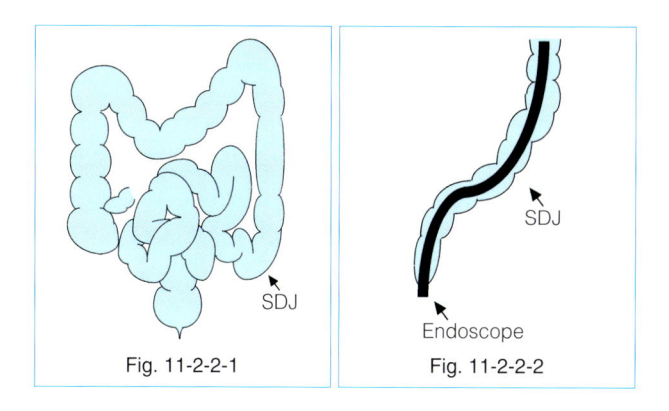

Fig. 11-2-2-1

Fig. 11-2-2-2

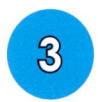

③ How to handle the case of dolichocolon (long colon)

Takahisa Matsuda

1. Things you can do to deal with dolichosigmoid

Long sigmoid colons may be found in patients who are tall and slender, patients who are elderly, or patients with a tendency to suffer from constipation. It is important to check the physical type and bowel habits of each patient before the examination.

Because of the elongation that occurs in dolichosigmoid cases, they often have more than one S-top. If a sigmoid colon has two S-tops, it forms an M-shaped loop. This means you must clear the second S-top after clearing the first. Therefore, it is important to clear every S-top using the insertion techniques described in other chapters (together with patient position change and hand pressure on the abdominal wall), while always assuming that there may be a second and even a third S-top.

In addition, being aware of the S-top is also important with an intestinal tract that forms an α-loop. If the intestinal lumen after the S-top goes straight or toward the left of the monitor screen, the existence of an α-loop can be predicted.

Once you have made this determination, advance the scope, being careful not to cause too much pain to the patient, and return to the N-loop just before an α-loop forms. Alternatively, leave the α-loop in place and release it after you have passed the SDJ. A certain degree of skill is required to perform the first technique successfully, while the second may facilitate smooth insertion when the patient position is changed to the right lateral position. However, an α-loop may cause pain to the patient because its formation temporarily stretches the intestinal tract excessively. If the patient complains about pain, we use an intravenous injection of a sedative or analgesic (35 mg of pethidine or 2-3 mg of midazolam).

2. Things you can do to deal with dolichotransversum

If you can insert the scope smoothly as far the splenic flexure but run into difficulty beyond that point, there are two possible explanations. One is deformation of the transverse colon, including the splenic flexure, due to adhesion after gastrectomy, and the other is dolichotransversum, which is elongation of the transverse colon.

In either case, the countermeasure is the same; insert the scope while keeping the scope shaft straight and use patient position changes and hand pressure appropriately. Since the transverse colon is highly mobile, it tends to sag like the sigmoid colon and stretches easily if the scope is pushed along the intestine. This is what is called the formation of a γ-loop. In this case, if you continue to advance the scope, not only will you cause pain to the patient, but the scope length will not be long enough to reach the cecum.

However, even in such a case, the basic insertion pattern remains the same. As already described in Chapter 9 ("Passing the Hepatic Flexure"), put the patient in the right lateral position and advance the scope to mid-T using the up-down slalom technique (while being careful to keep the scope shaft straight).

Normally, after mid-T is passed with counterclockwise rotation of the scope, pulling the scope while twisting it to the right causes it to approach the hepatic flexure. However, with a long transverse colon, another bend often exists. In this case, apply hand pressure to the abdominal wall to lift the umbilicus area upward so that the transverse colon does not sag and advance the scope by suctioning air.

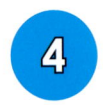

4 Countermeasures against dolichosigmoid

Osamu Tsuruta, Hiroshi Kawano

Generally, you can pass through a dolichosigmoid using similar insertion techniques to those you would use in sigmoid colons of normal lengths. In some cases, however, successful insertion requires the use of certain supplementary techniques. In this section, we will describe both the standard techniques we use with dolichosigmoid, as well as the supplementary techniques.

1. If double loops form

1) Remove the loop on the anal side before the loop on the oral side finishes forming:

When double loops are being formed, try to remove the loop on the anal side before the loop on the oral side has finished forming. Once you are sure you have passed the first loop before the loop on the oral side is fully formed, the trick is to pull the scope while twisting it in the direction in which the distal end stays in place.

2) Removing two loops one at a time (**Fig. 11-2-4-1**):

When double loops have already fully formed, remove the loop on the anal side first, then the one on the oral side. The loops on the anal and oral sides are often in opposite directions. After removing the loop on the anal side, immediately remove the one on the oral side by twisting the scope opposite to the way it was twisted to remove the anal-side loop with pulling of the scope. Make sure the scope's distal end stays in place.

3) Using a sliding tube:

When double loops have already fully formed and cannot be removed by any means and the scope's distal end cannot be advanced by pushing, it is recommended to use a sliding tube. Although this method is inconvenient because it should be performed under fluoroscopy, it is

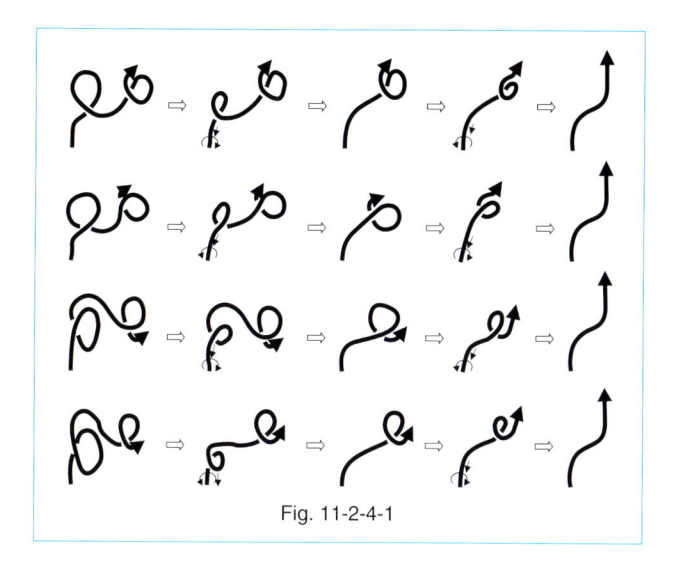

2) Dolichocolon (Sigmoid Colon, Transverse Colon)   167

Fig. 11-2-4-1

guaranteed to facilitate successful scope insertion. The trick is not to push in the scope all at once: Instead, insert the sliding tube little by little before any loops can form and advance slowly, taking advantage of the sliding tube's stiffness to prevent loop formation.

2. If a large loop has formed

This can occur with muscular or obese patients. In this case, a loop forms in the sigmoid colon and the scope's distal end cannot be advanced because simple pushing makes the loop bigger.

1) Apply hand pressure:

Pull the scope back to the rectum, and then compress strongly the suprapubic area in order to prevent loop formation. If a loop still forms, apply strong hand pressure to the area between the right lower abdomen and the right lateral region toward the pubic bone to prevent the loop from getting any bigger.

2) Using a thick, rigid scope:

Since an obese person has a large amount of adipose tissue in the mesentery, more force has to be applied to the scope in order to move the intestinal tract as desired. A thicker, more rigid scope is useful in this case because it can handle more force.

3) Using a sliding tube:

Loop formation can be minimized by the stiffness of the sliding tube.

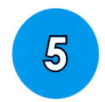

⑤ Ways to deal with dolichocolon cases

Satoru Tamura

1. Dolichosigmoid

Dolichosigmoid can be classified into the following two patterns.
① A long sigmoid colon that is folded into the pelvic cavity, forming numerous bends.
② A very long sigmoid colon that stretches to the proximity of the diaphragm without transverse folds being noticeable.

In the case of ①, the many bends in the sigmoid colon make it very difficult to pass the SD junction using a push-based insertion technique. Doing this also poses a risk of perforation, as well as causing pain. With such a case, hook the bend with the scope's distal end and pull the scope slightly, rotating it clockwise, while maintaining the angulation.

Counterclockwise rotation is sometimes required, but it is easier to control the scope, while monitoring the bend on the right of the screen and rotating the scope clockwise. Repeating this maneuver several times will eventually bring the scope to the SD junction.

If this maneuver is difficult with the patient in the left lateral position, you can try the supine or right lateral position. Occasionally, after successfully passing several bends, you may encounter a bend that cannot be hooked. As the sigmoid colon is already shortened and straightened to some extent in these cases, you should be able to reach the SD junction by pushing the scope and utilizing extra-abdominal pressure of hand as required. Once this procedure is accomplished, you should remove the loop and pass through the SD junction. Extra-abdominal pressure of an assistant's hand on the sigmoid colon is usually effective when the right lower abdomen is compressed after removing the loop in the sigmoid colon. Otherwise, extra-abdominal hand pressure is not only ineffective but also causes pain to the patient.

In the case of ②, it is hard to hook a bend with the scope's distal end even with the help of air suction and patient position change. With such a case, push the scope to the top of the sigmoid colon (bend), hook the bend with the distal end and pull back the scope to insert it as far as the SD junction as described above.

However, with a long pattern C sigmoid colon (2 in Chapter 6; page 79), it is often impossible to hook the bend properly with the scope's distal end. In this case, form a loop to prevent the walking-stick phenomenon, insert the scope deeper, then remove the loop to straighten the sigmoid colon and insert the scope until the SD junction.

With a long sigmoid colon, rotation of the scope with the right hand to remove the loop should be performed on a case-by-case basis. You should check the monitor image and the resistance felt by the right hand and manipulate the scope by confirming the angulation status and rotation direction so that the scope's distal end does not pull back toward the anal side.

2. Dolichotransverse

As the transverse colon protrudes toward the anterior wall in the abdominal cavity, the scope can be advanced as if pressing the intestinal tract toward the back by applying counterclockwise rotation. When the bend in the center of the transverse colon is passed, pull the scope while rotating it counterclockwise and suctioning air to reach the hepatic flexure. This method usually allows the scope to reach the hepatic flexure, but does not work in the following cases.

① **When there is difficulty clearing the bend in the center**: This often occurs when the scope's axis is deviated. When shortening and straightening are insufficient, the pushing force of the right hand is not transmitted to the distal end and a loop forms in the sigmoid colon. If this happens, withdraw the scope to the descending colon, straighten it completely and insert it again into the transverse colon.

It is also important to apply hand maneuver as required. If insertion past the bend is still not possible and the sigmoid colon is bended or the splenic flexure is bent like the handle of cane, try the right lateral position. This sometimes makes it possible to transmit the force of the right hand to the scope's distal end, allowing the scope to pass through the bend and reach the hepatic flexure with having to perform any more shortening operations.

② **If a γ-loop forms**: If the colon is not stretched too much and the cecum can be reached, observation can often be continued without removing it.

However, if the cecum cannot be reached even when the scope is inserted so deeply that the forceps port contacts the anal canal or if advanced scope control is necessary to treat a lesion, you will need to remove the loop. In this case, remove the loop with counterclockwise rotation if the scope was inserted with clockwise rotation, or with clockwise rotation if the scope was inserted with counterclockwise rotation.

11. How to Deal with Cases Where Insertion Is Difficult
3) Other

1 Advanced obesity cases

Sumio Tsuda

1. What insertion difficulties can advanced obesity cause?

In cases of advanced obesity cases where excessive adipose is deposited on the abdomen, the large amount of adipose surrounding the intestinal tract makes it difficult to shorten the tract and limits scope maneuverability. If it turns out that neither the sigmoid colon nor the transverse colon can be shortened sufficiently, the case can be considered a difficult insertion case, and will require an efficient combination of the push technique, hand pressure and patient position change to insert the scope.

2. Maneuvering the scope when using the push technique

If you try to advance the scope simply by pushing it, a repulsive force from the intestinal tract will prevent any forward movement. Pushing the scope in the sigmoid colon will do nothing but stretch the colon (direction of the arrow in **Fig. 11-3-1-1**).

Even when the scope reaches the splenic flexure, the scope cannot shorten the sigmoid colon completely, so, again, pushing it will succeed only in stretching the sigmoid colon (direction of arrow ♠ in **Fig. 11-3-1-2**). To avoid these problems, advance the scope as if pressing the intestinal tract with the scope shaft while twisting it clockwise. This technique is also applicable to insertion into the deeper part of the colon.

3. Hand pressure and patient position change

For insertion in the sigmoid colon, apply strong pressure to the right lower abdomen (★ in **Fig. 11-3-1-1**). During insertion into the deeper part of the colon after the splenic flexure, the intestinal tract deviates to the outer side (direction of arrow ♠ in **Fig. 11-3-1-2**), making it more difficult to advance the scope. In this case, compress the left abdomen towards the inner side, as well as applying pressure to the right lower abdomen (★ in **Fig. 11-3-1-2**). After the hepatic flexure, the hand pressure toward the inner side is to be applied to the right abdomen (★ in **Fig. 11-3-1-3**).

If the hand pressure on the right lower abdomen (★ in **Fig. 11-3-1-1**) is ineffective, change the patient position to the prone position. If this does not work, place a pillow below the patient's abdomen to apply pressure to it. In addition, also apply pressure to the left and right lateral regions as required.

4. Other measures

The most important thing is to combine scope maneuvers, hand pressure and patient position change as occasion may demand. However, suction of excessive air in the intestinal tract and utilization of the patient's breathing can often help insertion. The sliding tube and Variable Stiffness scope may also be useful, but there are also cases in which insertion is impossible unless a scope with a long working length is used.

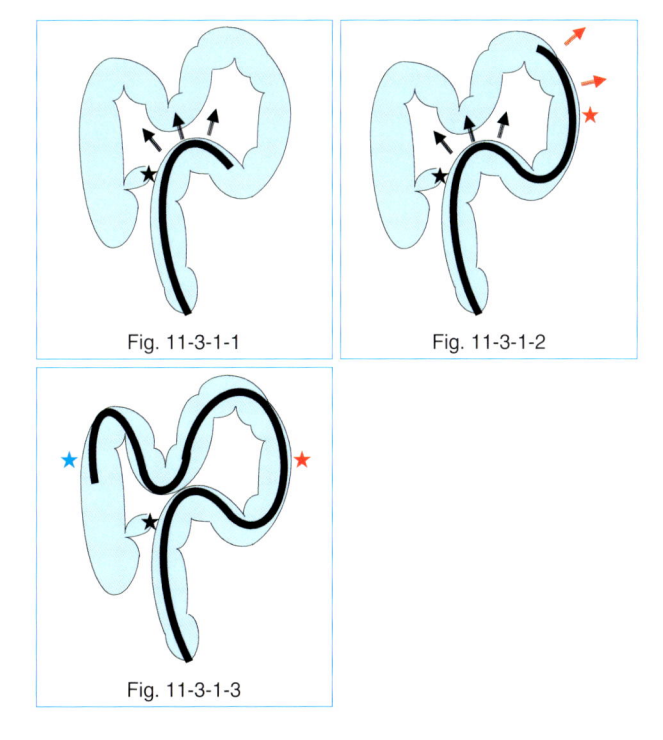

Fig. 11-3-1-1

Fig. 11-3-1-2

Fig. 11-3-1-3

② Patients undergoing pelvic radiation, patients with multiple sigmoid diverticula, thin women, elderly patients and patients with bloody stools

Norihiro Hamamoto

1. Use a slim scope in cases that have undergone pelvic radiation or with multiple sigmoid diverticula

Patients that have undergone pelvic radiation for uterine or prostate cancer often have strong adhesions in the pelvic region, making them typical examples of insertion difficulty. In addition, these cases have fragile mucosae due to the effects of radiation-induced colitis and the mucosal surfaces may bleed easily when touched by the scope's distal end.

Therefore, it is recommended to use a slim scope for insertion. In general, avoid contact with mucosal surfaces whenever possible, and insert the scope linearly. When the scope reaches the S-top, put the patient in the supine position. Ideally, advance the scope while pressing the pubic symphysis to prevent a loop from forming.

With cases that have multiple sigmoid diverticula, prediction of the orientation of the intestinal tract is difficult and peristalsis tends to occur easily. In addition, the presence of solid stool in the diverticula often makes insertion difficult. As the lumen has a narrow diameter and is spastic, the use of an antispasmodic is indispensable. To reduce the amount of stool left in the diverticula, it can be helpful to have the patient eat a low-residue diet the day before the examination.

As with cases of radiation colitis, a slim scope is also useful. Make sure you use utmost care when passing through each fold in order to avoid inserting the scope into a diverticulum. However, some cases do not have acute bends, so you can often advance the scope to the descending colon by performing a slight right turn in the SD junction.

2. A slim scope is also useful with thin women and elderly patients

Since thin women have narrow pelvic and abdominal cavities, very tight bends in the sigmoid colon can cause severe pain during insertion. Older patients, on the other hand, often have hardened colon walls so the risk of accidents such as perforation is higher than with younger patients. Older patients also tend to be thin, so the same sort of care is required as for thin women. In both cases, it is generally best to use a slim scope, to minimize the amount of air, and to insert the scope linearly.

3. Emergency colonoscopy for bloody stool

In emergency colonoscopy due to lower gastrointestinal bleeding, the necessity of identifying the bleeding source prevents the administration of colonic irrigation fluid and high-pressure enema. Instead, it is sometimes necessary to use a glycerin enema only or insert the scope without preparation.

Although high-pressure enema and colonic irrigation fluid can help ease insertion, they are not desirable in situations where identification of the bleeding source is the first priority. This naturally means that the scope has to be inserted under unfavorable conditions in the presence of blood clots. In such a case, a thick scope with a large suction channel should be used.

Advance the scope slowly as far as the descending colon, using repeated irrigation and suction, while watching for the subsequent lumen. If the segment as far the sigmoid colon can be rinsed sufficiently, the scope slides well and will be able to reach the cecum smoothly.

If rinsing cannot remove the attached stool, it may be necessary to start over, possibly using a high-pressure enema. However, once the scope reaches the splenic flexure, the lumen becomes wider and it is possible to insert it deeper by pushing through the blood clots.

③ Dealing with adhesions, patients whose position cannot be changed, transverse colon loops, sigmoid colon volvulus and melena

Eisai Cho

1. Cases with adhesion

Insertion is often difficult in patients who have undergone surgery in the lower abdomen, particularly after surgery of appendicitis accompanied with peritonitis, uterine/ovarian surgery or exposure to irradiation, as well as strictures of diverticulosis and repeated inflammations.

With a case that has undergone lower abdominal surgery, insertion gets more difficult depending on how complicated the adhesion is — from partial to extensive adhesion or adhesions between intestinal tracts.

With a case with diverticulosis, the lumen is narrower and mobility is degraded so the scope cannot be adjusted correctly for shortening and twisting. As the twisting maneuver is less effective than normal, it is necessary to angulate the scope more frequently to the left and right. As a stiffer or thicker scope is hard to maneuver and causes pain easily, it is recommended to use a pliant or slim scope.

2. Cases where position change is not possible

In normal cases, patient position change is an effective way to facilitate insertion. However, some patients cannot change position or breathe deeply. In such cases, it is also necessary to prepare and attach a sliding tube to the scope before insertion.

3. Cases with loop in the transverse colon

When a loop forms in the transverse colon, it makes insertion into the cecum difficult. If the loop cannot be removed by shortening and straightening, it is easier to remove the loop after having inserted the scope into the cecum by stretching the colon. The loop can be eliminated by clockwise or counterclockwise twisting. From the endoscopist's perspective, removal of a loop in the transverse colon seems to require more forceful twisting and to take longer than that required for the removal of a loop in the sigmoid colon.

4. Cases with sigmoid colon volvulus

With cases with sigmoid colon volvulus, the sigmoid colon is remarkably twisted and enlarged by intestinal gas. Preparation is ineffective and insertion is often extremely difficult. Since the purpose of this operation is restoration, the scope does not have to be inserted beyond the descending or transverse colon. Instead, what is required is to shorten and straighten the sigmoid colon and suction the intestinal gas to prevent recurrence of the volvulus. It is recommended to use a long scope attached with a long sliding tube. Because of the difficulty of insertion, the necessity of checking the intestinal gas condition and the high probability of erroneous recognition of the distal-end positions of the scope and sliding tube, it is desirable to combine fluoroscopy with insertion.

5. Cases with melena

Colonoscopy of cases with melena is sometimes performed without preparation. As the intestinal tract is filled with fresh blood or blood clots attached to the intestinal walls, it is as dark as a cave and visibility is low.

If a blood clot gets on the front lens of the scope's distal end, vision is even more obscured, hindering insertion. To deal with this, it is necessary to irrigate the colon frequently with water using the irrigation nozzle or biopsy channel in order to wash the lens surface and intestinal wall.

Inevitably, this will increase insufflation, making insertion even more difficult. When inserting the scope in such a case, determine the orientation of the lumen, keeping your eyes open for any glimpses of the lumen.

It is sometimes necessary to change the patient position to move the blood-accumulated region and find the orientation of the lumen. Poor visibility inside the lumen makes quick insertion almost impossible, and you will have to be patient and persistent.

12. Examining Elderly Patients (80 or Older)

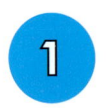

1 Caution is required for insertion in elderly patients

Yuji Inoue

1. Causes of insertion difficulties in elderly patients (80 or older)

While many older people today are robust enough to withstand normal insertion techniques, quite a few still present the endoscopist with insertion difficulties.

The main causes of these difficulties include ① poor preparation, ② poor intestinal tract mobility due to adhesions and ③ low physical resistance to invasive procedures such as scope insertion. Moreover, the frequency of cases with insertion difficulties increases as the age of the patients increases. I measure the time taken for insertion for reference data for the subsequent examinations, classifying cases where insertion takes less than 3 minutes as "very easy", those taking 3 minutes to 4 minutes and 30 seconds as "easy", those taking 4 minutes and 30 seconds up to 7 minutes as "medium", and those taking 7 minutes or more as "difficult".

"Medium" cases are categorized as requiring care, because they include cases that were originally "easy" but took time because mistakes were made and those that were originally "difficult" but took less time because insertion was able to be done very smoothly.

The other day, I examined an 84-year-old woman, who undergoes colonoscopy every year because of a history of colon polypectomy. She has also a history of distal pancreatectomy due to a pancreatic tumor, so her colon has some adhesions. As her last exam took exactly 7 minutes, I proceeded with the exam cautiously, assuming that she might be a "medium" or "difficult" case.

The insertion in the shortening technique succeeded with almost no pain and took 6 minutes and 40 seconds. I was pleased to have inserted the scope almost perfectly in less time than previously. However, when I reviewed the examination history in her medical chart, I found that the time taken in previous examinations was even less — exactly 5 minutes in the exam before the last one, 4.5 minutes in the examination before that, and between 3 and 4 minutes in the two preceding examinations. All of the exams were done without sedation.

While my skill was established five or six years ago, I believe it has improved a little since then. Some cases can be inserted quickly mainly by pushing the scope using the loop formation technique. But this woman had adhesions that necessitated the shortening technique for pain-free insertion. Naturally, this patient had not undergone a laparotomy since she started undergoing colonoscopy. This case forced me to reconfirm the need for caution in scope insertion in elderly patients.

2. Countermeasures against causes of insertion difficulties

1) Poor preparation

Preparation is often poor with elderly patients. The causes include an increased tendency for age-related constipation and the difficulty of taking a full dose of Niflec® or the like within two or three hours.

A good countermeasure against this is to administer premedication. I usually prescribe one or two bottles of Laxoberon® to be taken before bedtime the day before the examination. This results in extensive bowel movement in the morning, sometimes making it possible to reduce the Niflec® dose.

If this still does not make the examination easier, it is also recommended that the patient be given the same diet used in preparation for a barium enema examination.

2) Poor intestinal tract mobility due to adhesions

This makes it indispensable to master insertion using the shortening technique. Adhesions are not uncommon among older persons even when they have never undergone a laparotomy. With these cases, the scope should be inserted by folding the intestinal tract without forming a loop, while taking maximum care to avoid causing pain.

3) Low physical resistance against invasive procedures such as scope insertion
This can be dealt with in a similar manner to 2) above. In our center, we experienced a case in which excessive stretching produced during insertion with an elderly patient caused a shock due to vagal reflex.

To prevent an accident, it is important to observe the patient carefully during the procedure. The fragility of the intestinal wall should also be considered. As the probability of perforation due to excessive stretching is expected to be higher than in a normal case, a high degree of caution is required for insertion.

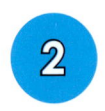

② Watch out for any changes in vital signs

Yasumoto Suzuki

1. Precautions when examining elderly patients (80 or older)

Total colonoscopy (TCS) on patients aged 80 or older require you to pay special attention to any changes in vital signs. Even a small change that a younger patient could easily recover from can develop into a serious problem with an elderly patient.

Safety should always be your first priority in TCS. In this section, I will describe the various precautions you should take when performing TCS on elderly persons.

2. Preparation

There is no method of preparation used exclusively for older patients. However, while lavage of the intestinal tract with the goal of eliminating all residue is emphasized in standard preparation, the most important thing to focus on when prepping older patients is to make sure there is no deterioration of vital signs.

With elderly patients receiving TCS for the first time, I ask them if they have any tendency to constipation. Patients who have or are suspected to have a tendency to constipation are prepared using the modified Brown's method in place of intestinal lavage.

3. Sedation

I reduce the amount of sedative used with patients over 70, reducing it even further for those aged 80 or more. In some cases, sedation is omitted altogether with patients over 80 years or older, depending on comorbidities and body weight.

4. Insertion method

As with preparation, there is no special insertion method for use with older patients. However, I always try to be more sensitive to changes in intestinal tract resistance sensed by the right hand during scope maneuvers.

I am also more cautious when performing scope maneuvers that usually produce only weak resistance, such as pushing, pulling or turning the scope. Even if it means it takes longer to perform the procedure, I always manipulate the scope slowly and carefully in fine increments, avoiding any big or sudden maneuvers.

In their determination to reach the cecum, some endoscopists tend to execute riskier scope maneuvers. However, care is required with older patients because a slightly forced maneuver that would usually work may cause a serious problem. Regardless of the circumstances, the key to safe TCS is being able to properly determine whether or not TCS is possible and being willing to discontinue TCS if necessary.

5. Recovery

I usually wake up patients 45 minutes after sedation, but wait at least an hour with elderly patients.

③ The importance of avoiding risks and knowing when to stop

Hiroyuki Tsukagoshi

Since the intestinal tracts of elderly persons are delicate and more prone to bleeding and perforation, it is important to never take any unnecessary risks and to be prepared to stop the examination in the event of strong resistance. In this section, I will discuss the best methods of preparation, sedation and insertion when performing colonoscopy on elderly patients.

1. Preparation

Preparation can lead to ileus or perforation if a severe stricture is present. With a new elderly outpatient, useful information can usually be obtained by examining only the visible regions such as the rectum and sigmoid colon after natural bowel movement without the application of any preparation.

In many cases, insertion into the deeper part of the colon is possible without preparation. If necessary, a total colonoscopy can be performed after preparation on another day. In this case the patient may need hospitalization depending on their condition.

2. Sedation

As a general rule, sedation is not administered to patients aged 75 or older. If a patient requests sedation, the dosage should be half the usual. Since many older patients have heart and/or respiratory system complications or poor hepatic and/or renal functioning, their blood pressure and oxygen partial pressure should be monitored at all times, with special attention given to their breathing condition.

It is also important to be careful when changing the patient position, as the supine position may cause cyanosis due to depression of the tongue root. When the endoscopy suite is not very bright, it is difficult to detect cyanosis early, making it necessary to check the breathing on a regular basis. First-aid tools such as airway and tracheal intubation tubes should also be kept handy.

3. Insertion method

When examining an older person with poor general status, a slim scope should be used. If resistance is felt, do not push the scope with force; instead, use patient position change and hand pressure.

The most important factor is the amount of air. If the scope can be inserted by slowly pushing its way through the mucosa while insufflating as little air as possible, an examination can be performed with perfect safety and absence of pain.

The most important point to be noted in the insertion technique is the clearance between the intestinal wall and scope. Keep the scope a few millimeters from the intestinal wall, align the direction and angle of each curve, and pull back the scope to open the subsequent lumen in a narrow space that is almost closed. The key to the success is to manipulate the scope as slowly as possible.

4. Knowing when to stop

When insertion difficulties are encountered, regardless of whether the patient is elderly or not, be especially careful not to insufflate too much air and make full use of patient position change and hand pressure. If the scope still cannot be inserted, the last resort is to push it. However, as this presents a risk of perforation, be prepared to discontinue the examination and switch to a barium enema examination.

4 Elderly patients usually have more fragile colons

Shinji Tanaka

1. Recognize the correct physical age of each patient

This section deals with the precautions that need to be taken when performing colonoscopies on patients aged 80 or older. Even among the elderly, the actual chronological age and the physical age often do not correspond. It is important to accurately estimate the physical age of each patient, as this will help determine whether the colonoscopy is really necessary.

2. Be sure to obtain accurate clinical and medication histories

Elderly patients often have coexisting diseases, so it is important to make sure you obtain detailed and accurate clinical and medication histories. Preparation with intestinal lavage can sometimes put excessive stress on the patient, so care has to be taken not to do anything that might induce or aggravate ischemic heart diseases.

Specifically, when a patient takes coronary vasodilators and/or antihypertensive drugs, make sure they take them on the morning of the examination as usual. Considering that the patient will have fasted for a half or full day before the examination, it may be necessary to rehydrate the patient before and after the examination in order to prevent organ ischemia (angina, cerebral infarction, ischemic enteritis, renal failure, etc.) due to dehydration.

Caution is also required against careless premedication or sedation as this could induce respiratory arrest. If a sedative is administered, it is essential to prepare the antagonist drug and monitor the patient until they have recovered sufficiently.

3. Colonoscopy precautions

In actual colonoscopy of elderly patients, you have to be extremely careful when maneuvering the scope because of the thinness of the colonic walls. Because the muscular layer of the colon in elderly patients has often atrophied, any forceful scope maneuver could easily perforate the colon. Forced insertion or excessive air insufflation during examination may also lead to ischemic enteritis after examination.

Older persons are sometimes slow to react to pain, so you have to be careful here as well. While these precautions are not limited to the elderly, of course, it is of paramount importance to perform gentle, low-impact, gentle examinations on elderly persons.

⑤ Key points when examining patients aged 80 or older

Yusuke Saitoh

Key points
- Determine if the indications for colonoscopy are optimum. Before examination, check whether the patient has any complications anywhere else in the body, takes anticoagulants, or has chronic constipation.
- Serious side effects of sedation, such as respiratory depression or a drop in blood pressure, manifest particularly easily with elderly persons. Keep the use of sedation to a minimum.
- Perform the procedure cautiously and be prepared to stop immediately at the slightest sign of trouble.
- Select the scope according to the physique of the patient. Use a thin scope or Variable Stiffness scope as required.

When examining elderly patients, always be prepared to deal with unpredictable events, which occur more frequently than with younger adult patients. When an endoscopist is asked to examine an elderly patient, the first thing that should be done is to determine whether or not the indications for colonoscopy are optimal.

Before examination, be sure to check for existing complications, including the respiratory, circulatory and renal functions. Also check whether the patient takes anticoagulants or has chronic constipation. If a biopsy or endoscopic treatment is considered necessary, the anticoagulant should be stopped beforehand if possible.

Complications with elderly patients can be categorized into two basic groups: those caused by preparation or sedation; and those resulting from procedure techniques. Preparation-related complications that can be induced include death by lavage solution in elderly patients with chronic constipation, so it is important to inquire about bowel movements in the pre-examination interview.

For patients with chronic constipation, laxatives and a bowel motility stimulant a few days before the examination will be recommended. In addition, since older patients are often unable to drink all of the whole gut lavage fluid, the use of a bowel cleansing method with small amount of load fluid such as the Magcorol® or Laxoberon® should be considered in place of the polyethylene glycol solution lavage.

As many elderly patients are also very thin and frail, premedication can cause serious side effects such as respiratory depression or a sudden drop in blood pressure, particularly in cases where sedation is necessary. If sedation is used, start with a very small amount and keep the total dose to a minimum. Even when an antagonist is administered after the examination, unexpected incidents, such as a fall, can occur afterwards, so a family member should be asked to be on hand to assist the post-examination patient whenever possible.

Because so many elderly patients are very thin, they tend to have long intestinal tracts, making examinations more difficult. In addition, the fragility of mucosae and walls of the intestinal tract could lead to unexpected complications.

I have experienced some frightening moments, including bleeding from a long mucosal rupture near the splenic flexure despite the fact that the examination was performed very cautiously and the scope was inserted as far as the cecum with no problem (nor complaint of pain from the patient whatsoever).

In case of insertion difficulty with an elderly patient, the same countermeasures described in my previous article (1-5 in Chapter 11; page 156) are required. Namely, perform the procedure cautiously, never take any unnecessary risks, be prepared to stop at the first sign of difficulty. Use a thin, flexible scope with a diameter of around 10 mm or less, or a scope with the Variable Stiffness function.

13. Preventing Perforation during Insertion

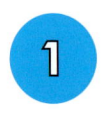

① Do not use force to manipulate the scope

Yasumoto Suzuki

1. The cause of perforation during insertion

It is no exaggeration to say that perforations during scope insertion are caused almost exclusively by the use of too much force when manipulating the scope. The question, then, is in what situations do colonoscopists tend to use too much force?

Here is an interesting fact: Among all the colonoscopists at our facilities — from novices with almost no experience to "super"-class experts — the ones who most commonly cause perforations are those at the intermediate level. The next question is, why do intermediate colonoscopists cause so many perforations, while novices, beginners and experts do not?

Novices and beginners rarely cause perforations because they handle the scope very carefully and slowly, having no idea at what point the examination might enter the danger zone. Experts, on the other hand, seldom cause perforations because they manipulate the scope knowing exactly where the limits of safety are.

However, when a colonoscopist moves from the novice level to the intermediate level, they tend to become overly confident in their ability to manipulate the scope, taking unnecessary chances and using too much force, thereby increasing the risk of perforation.

2. Unnecessary scope manipulation

Now, what sorts of maneuvers that could be regarded as unnecessary are typically attempted by mid-level colonoscopists? The most common is the application of force in the direction where increased resistance has been felt with the right hand holding the scope.

For instance, there are times when resistance is felt and the image on the monitor does not move at all and turns red when the scope is pushed. This happens when the scope's distal end is perpendicularly in contact with the intestinal mucosa. In this situation, continuing to push the scope increases the risk of perforation.

There are also times when pulling or turning the scope is difficult due to resistance. This is because the scope is being moved in a direction that would severely twist the intestinal tract. If the colonoscopist keeps trying to pull or turn the scope in this situation, the risk of perforation increases significantly.

3. Prevention of perforation during insertion

Most perforations can be prevented by avoiding the sorts of unnecessary scope manipulations described above. The key to preventing perforations is to be aware of the resistance felt by the right hand holding the scope.

On the other hand, being too concerned about any resistance can result in the colonoscopist being afraid to move the scope even when minimal resistance is felt, making it impossible to perform TCS smoothly. Therefore, the key to mastering TCS without the risk of perforation is to learn under the guidance of an instructor early on at what level of resistance it is safe to continue moving the scope.

② Always perform insertion carefully and be prepared to discontinue the procedure before completion

Hiroyuki Tsukagoshi

1. Causes of perforation

Accidental perforation occurs at our hospital about once every 10,000 procedures. These incidents are not always caused by beginners. In fact, they are more likely to happen when an endoscopist has begun to gain confidence in their ability — usually after having experience in about 1,000 cases or so.

While perforations can be caused by problems with the patient's physical condition such as adhesions formed during laparotomy, endoscopists who have caused perforations often report that they do not know why the perforations occurred and that they did not apply so much force. They seem puzzled that the perforation occurred with a specific patient, even though there are many cases where they have applied much greater force when pushing the scope.

Personally, I have never caused a perforation during insertion. In my opinion, the intestinal tract is very tough, rarely suffering damage even when the scope is pushed with a fairly strong force. Even so, it seems that the scope's distal end turns into a blade at the most unexpected moments.

When a perforation occurs, those involved usually report that the hole was opened very easily. Therefore, when examining a patient with poor whole body status or an elderly patient, it is safer to assume that the patient has a very fragile intestinal tract.

Perforation rarely occurs if the scope is inserted correctly using a small amount of air. Since pushing the scope turns the monitor image completely red, making observation impossible, always keep the distance between the scope and intestinal wall at 1 or 2 mm and manipulate the scope slowly while advancing it. This will make you feel more confident, while ensuring that the patient is not subjected to unnecessary pain.

2. If insertion is difficult

Once in a while — every few hundred cases or so — insertion will be difficult regardless of what you do. If the scope cannot be inserted, the last resort is to push it in.

I always have two scopes handy — a thick, stiff one and a slim, flexible one. Normally, I use the thick scope but, whenever I feel strong resistance or the patient complains of pain, I immediately replace the thick scope with the thin one and start over from the beginning. It is also important to know how to use the patient position change and hand pressure appropriately.

Beginners who sense strong resistance during procedure should discontinue it immediately or have a skilled endoscopist perform it. Should a perforation occur, it not only spoils the examination but may result in a medical lawsuit, which is an unpleasant experience for both the endoscopist and patient.

③ The importance of identifying high-risk cases

Norihiro Hamamoto

Unlike other types of endoscopic examination, colonoscopy is accompanied with the risk of perforation in the action of insertion itself. Perforation during insertion typically starts not with the mucosa, but with the muscle layer. As the mucosa is the last layer of tissue to be perforated, it is almost impossible to predict it from the lumen side.

When force is used to push or angulate a scope in a bend, the monitor image will turn completely red. Continuing to push will result in the distal end of the scope perforating the intestine.

Also, if a large loop is formed and removed carelessly, the distal end might disengage and the resulting bounce-back of the shaft could produce a big rupture on the mucosa side. In addition, when the intestinal tract is overly stretched because there is too much air, even ordinary scope manipulation could cause a perforation.

This risk increases even more with a case accompanied with intestinal adhesion. In almost all cases, severe abdominal pain caused by excessive stretching of the intestinal tract due to scope pushing is observed before the occurrence of perforation.

1. Make sure to conduct a full interview and consultation before the examination

Perforations rarely occur during the screening examination of a healthy individual. The frequency of perforation tends to increase among high-risk patients such as those with intestinal adhesion or those who are elderly. Potential high-risk cases without subjective symptoms also exist — sub-ileus cases, for example.

It is imperative that a detailed interview and consultation be conducted in order to identify whether the indication for colonoscopy is accurate and, if necessary, to obtain a plain radiograph of the abdomen before examination. The abdominal examination should always be performed immediately before the colonoscopic examination.

2. Observe the basic rules of insertion

The basic rules of insertion refer to use of the technique of shortening the colonic fold through bending" to advance the scope linearly, while keeping the intestinal tract permanently collapsed. If the patient complains of pain or if resistance is felt when pushing the scope, pull back the scope and retry approach. If you stick to these rules at all times, the risk of perforation will be virtually eliminated.

If insertion is not possible, regardless of what method you try, you should go back as far as the rectum and retry your approach from there. Naturally, meticulous care is required with the cases which present a higher risk of perforation than ordinary patients, such as patients with advanced adhesion due to laparotomy or cancerous peritonitis, patients with multiple sigmoid diverticulums and elderly patients.

Inadvertent use of a sedative or analgesic should be avoided because they can obscure signs that would normally warn us that the patient is at risk of intestinal tract perforation.

3. Always be prepared to discontinue the procedure if necessary

No endoscopist, regardless of skill level, is immune from the risk of perforation by insertion, so you always need to be alert to any situation that could cause perforation. Special caution is required if you find yourself feeling frustrated or impatient because the insertion cannot be done as planned. If a novice or beginner-level endoscopist is unable to successfully pass through a given region after trying for 10 to 15 minutes, they should be replaced with a more experienced endoscopist.

Insertion problems are not restricted to beginners, however. Even intermediate or expert endoscopists encounter occasionally experience insertion difficulty. If this happens and the endoscopist is unable to work the scope through a particular region, even after trying all possible insertion patterns and support techniques, or if the patient complains of continuous pain, the right thing to do is discontinue the insertion and cancel the procedure.

④ Avoid applying excessive force to the colon wall

Sumio Tsuda

1. Causes of perforation during scope insertion

It is well known that applying excessive force to the colon wall with a scope increases the risk of perforation. This includes direct force from the scope's distal end and shaft and indirect force produced when the scope is manipulated. Here are some techniques you can use to avoid applying excessive force to the colon walls in order to prevent perforation.

2. How to avoid applying direct force to the colon wall

If the monitor image is completely red with no sign of the lumen at all or if the observed mucosal surface looks dry, it means that the scope's distal end is in close contact with the mucosa. Continuing to push the scope in this situation will increase the acuteness of the angle formed by the colon wall and distal end, thereby increasing the pressure on the colon wall, causing perforation.

To avoid perforation, pull the scope back until the lumen is visible and then reinsert it. One of the rules of scope insertion is to constantly check the lumen during insertion. This rule should be observed under all circumstances.

Sometimes you will find that the scope will not advance any further when pushed. Using force to advance the scope in this case will result in excessive force being applied to the colon wall by the scope shaft, risking perforation. If the scope cannot be advanced by pushing, do not use force; instead, try applying hand pressure or patient position change. Also be sure to use a slim scope when using the push technique as this will apply less force to the colon wall.

3. How to avoid applying indirect force to the colon wall

When the scope is inserted in the wrong direction or when there is an adhesion, the intestinal tract may look twisted when viewed on the monitor. If the scope is pushed to advance into the twisted region, excessive force is applied indirectly to the twisted or adhered region, causing a risk of perforation.

If strong resistance is felt by the right hand manipulating the scope or if the scope cannot be angulated or moved due to strong resistance, it means that the scope is stuck in the intestinal tract — an extremely dangerous situation. To eliminate the danger, the scope should be withdrawn promptly whenever the intestinal tract is twisted. After withdrawal, retry insertion using a technique that will not twist the intestinal tract, such as changing the insertion direction or using hand pressure.

If the colon has an adhesion, indirect force can be applied to the colon wall not only by pushing, but also by using the shortening maneuver. This is especially so when the maneuver is performed quickly, rapidly shortening the intestinal tract and increasing the force applied to the adhered region as well as the risk of perforation. Therefore, it is important to always manipulate the scope slowly.

⑤ Situations where perforation can occur and how to avoid them

Masahiro Igarashi

In general, perforation during insertion is caused by forceful pushing or manipulation of the scope. In this section, we will look at the situations in which perforation can occur and discuss ways to prevent it.

1. When scope control is difficult
When it is difficult to angulate the scope or move the shaft because the scope is stuck, this can be the result of non-physiological force applied due to a complicated loop or excessive stretching of the intestinal tract. If this happens, do not try unreasonable procedure; instead, return the angulation to the neutral state, withdraw the scope until there is no more resistance, and then try again.

2. When the image shown during contact with the mucosa (completely red) cannot be moved
You can safely change scope angulation while the monitor image is completely red, as long as you can move the scope's distal end or, when pushing the scope, the imaged mucosa smoothly. If you feel any resistance or if smooth movement is not possible, do not try to use force to push the scope as this could cause a laceration or perforation of the mucosa. When the monitor image of the mucosa turns completely red and cannot be moved smoothly, it is necessary to withdraw the scope until the lumen is visible and retry insertion.

3. When removing the loop
If you twist the scope forcefully against high resistance to remove the loop, it will stretch the mucosa excessively, increasing the risk of perforation. Do not twist a scope in any direction where you feel resistance.
<Is pain a sign of perforation?>
Even when the patient experiences some pain during insertion, the

endoscopist usually continues with the procedure anyway. However, if the cause of pain cannot be identified or if the patient complains strongly about pain, it is necessary to discontinue the procedure and retry insertion from the beginning. It takes a lot of experience before an endoscopist is capable of judging whether the patient's pain is dangerous or not. If the patient experiences pain while you are performing a procedure, you must be willing to admit that that pain is a manifestation of your own lack of skill. If you determine that the case difficulty requires more skill than you can offer, you need to have the courage to promptly discontinue the procedure.

4. When the patient complains of pain after the procedure
Post-procedural pain is often caused by residual air. This pain can often be reduced by "degassing" the colon. You can do this by inserting a Nelaton catheter from the anus and changing the patient's position. However, if the patient complains of severe pain, take an x-ray of the abdomen and check for perforations. Sending the patient home without doing anything can result in major problems if a complication subsequently occurs as a result of the examination.

5. Things to keep in mind in order to avoid perforation
① Do not use excessive force to push the scope.
② Insert the scope gently and slowly.
③ Know the limits of your own skill.
④ Remember that colonoscopy is not the only examination method available.
⑤ If a skilled endoscopist is available, call and seek advice.

6. Cautions on use of sedative and analgesic
As patients under sedation do not normally complain of pain, you will not be able to rely on this as a means of assessing risk. You will need to literally feel it with your hand. If the scope seems stuck or you feel significant resistance, this should tell you that further scope manipulation is risky.

⑥ When caution is required during insertion

Yuji Inoue

Avoiding perforation is of critical importance during colonoscopic insertion. Fortunately, its frequency is rather rare. In this section, I will discuss some examples of perforation during insertion that occurred at our facilities recently.

1. Perforation in the vicinity of SD junction

In one case, perforation was caused when a beginner pushed the scope excessively. A situation like this can occur when an endoscopist pushes the scope without being able to see the lumen on the front near the SD junction. As a result, a laparoscopist must be called in to remedy the situation.

Here, it should be emphasized that the technique of sliding the scope by guessing where the lumen is when it cannot be observed (slide-by-the-mucosa technique) should be avoided whenever possible — even by experienced endoscopists. If loop formation is unavoidable, always insert the scope using counterclockwise rotation to ensure that an α-loop is formed. Obtaining a frontal view of the lumen may not be possible in this case, so position the opposite side of the bend in the 6 o'clock direction of the image and insert the scope cautiously using upward angulation.

2. Example of multiple sigmoid diverticulums

Caution is also required with a case with multiple sigmoid diverticulums. In one case, a mid-level endoscopist with 7 or 8 years of experience was inserting a scope from the rectum into the sigmoid colon (near the RS junction) when the view was momentarily lost; the endoscopist then pushed the scope slightly and this produced a perforation.

He was fairly skilled and said he did not push the scope too much.

The perforation may have occurred because the scope accidentally entered a fragile section of the diverticulum. This underlines the danger of insertion in cases with multiple sigmoid diverticula.

3. Adhesion

Postoperative adhesions can present particular difficulties. If the patient complains of pain during insertion, you must be extra cautious. Even when sedation is used, you can still get a rough idea of the amount of pain being experienced by observing the patient's body movements.

I myself experienced perforation during insertion two years ago. The patient initially had sigmoid colon carcinoma with synchronous hepatic metastasis and received sigmoidectomy and partial hepatectomy. Subsequently, the patient underwent two hepatectomy operations (extended resection of the right hepatic lobe and partial hepatectomy) due to metachronous hepatic metastases. When we saw the patient, he had survived without recurrence for six years since the last hepatectomy.

I had been examining the patient every year using sedation because of the difficulty of insertion from the transverse colon to the ascending colon perhaps due to the adhesion of transverse colon to the hepatectomized surface. The examination findings of this patient also included a note saying that insertion from transverse colon to the ascending colon was performed with push operation.

On the day of examination two years ago, we used a new scope that had just been introduced. Perhaps because this scope was stiff, a perforation was made during insertion and free air was observed in a broad area on the next day. The scope was inserted as far as the cecum in the examination, and no mucosal injury was observed during the scope withdrawal. However, abdominal distension appeared after the patient was awakened using an antagonist. Although free air was recognized, the problem was solved by conservative management, perhaps because the patient was a poly-surgery case. The patient left the hospital in a week.

Unlike post-EMR perforations that are often of the pinhole type, perforations made by insertion generally consist of ruptures of all layers and necessitate surgical resections. There was even a case where perforation was made the day after a pain-free total colonoscopy performed six months after a fundectomy involved with the transverse colon interposition (the perforation was made because the adhesion in the colon and the anastomotic region of the colon was separated).

Incidentally, I supervised the latter case from beginning to end, but have no memory of any problems during the procedure. During the examination of a peritoneal disseminated metastasis, there was an instance of perforation in the middle of almost resistance-free, perhaps because of a cancerous adhesion. Both this case and the previous case required laparotomy. As a large amount of ascitic fluid was observed with the latter case, it is possible that the case should not have been indicated for colonoscopy.

14. Observation Tips

1 When is the best time for observation?

Yasumoto Suzuki

1. During insertion or during withdrawal?

In about 1980 when I began performing total colonoscopies (TCS), we generally made our observations during scope insertion. The reason we did this was because the scopes in those days had long bending sections which could not be bent sharply, making it difficult to observe the oral sides of the folds during withdrawal.

Today's scopes have shorter, more acutely bendable bending sections, so observations are made during insertion, as well as during withdrawal. This is to minimize the chance of missing any lesions since the appearance of the intestinal tract differs during insertion and withdrawal. However, spending too much time making detailed observations during scope insertion can make insertion difficult, so I usually do it during scope withdrawal.

2. Observation method

Performing observations exclusively during scope withdrawal increases the chances of not detecting lesions. This is because the oral sides of the folds are hidden from view during withdrawal.

To overcome this problem, I withdraw the scope by repeatedly pulling back a little and then returning a little. This is a kind of reciprocatory observation, in which I observe the oral side of each fold by flipping it during pullback and the anal side of the fold during when the scope goes back in.

This reciprocatory observation will permit observation during insertion, making it possible to significantly reduce dead spots and minimize the risk of missing lesions. The key to reciprocatory observation is persistence. Having the persistence to review the same region several times whenever observation is insufficient or a lesion is suspected is an essential characteristic for endoscopists.

3. Residual fluids and bubbles
Residual fluids including lavage and enema fluids and watery stools should be suctioned as much as possible. Spray Gascon® solution if bubbles are present so you do not miss any lesions hidden below the residual fluids and bubbles. This is necessary because unexpectedly large lesions are sometimes hidden beneath. On a number of occasions, I have discovered laterally spreading tumors (LSTs) as large as 15 to 20 cm hidden beneath bubbles.

4. Insufflation and deaeration
Proper observation inside the intestinal tract is not possible unless the tract is dilated to some extent by insufflating air. Unnecessary air is naturally deaerated after observation, but some patients complain about strong abdominal distension due to insufficient deaeration.

If I know that there is a high probability of abdominal distension with the current patient or situation, I do not end the colonoscopy after observation as far the rectum. Instead, I re-insert the scope to the cecum and then withdraw it while focusing exclusively on deaeration. This takes time, but is much simpler than having the patient complain about strong distension at rest for a long period.

② Observation by withdrawing the scope a little at a time

Masahiro Igarashi

The basic observation technique is to begin observation after reaching the cecum and to observe the full circumference of the intestinal tract by maneuvering the scope as if drawing a circle with the distal end while pulling it out slowly, a little at a time. During observation, insufflate some air to dilate the lumen. Keep the following points in mind regarding colon observation.

1. Use an anticholinergic agent for observation

The anticholinergic agent is useful for observation. I inject Buscopan® (1 A) intramuscularly immediately before insertion. If the scope can be inserted as far as the cecum in a few minutes, this is exactly when the drug begins to manifest the effect, which is very convenient for observation. The anticholinergic agent cannot be used with cases for which it is contraindicated (prostatic hyperplasia, cardiac diseases, glaucoma, etc.).

2. Use retroflexed observation in the right-side colon

In the right-side colon which has strong haustra, the back of the crescentic folds tend to be hidden from observation. To observe them, it helps to retroflex the tip of the scope at the cecum. The scope tip can be retroflexed by angulating the scope up or down in the cecum as far as it will go and pushing gently. When the scope comes into view on the monitor, withdraw the scope while twisting the shaft clockwise or counterclockwise to observe the whole ascending colon. To return the retroflexed scope tip to the original orientation, neutralize the angulation and pull the scope.

3. Put the region to be observed in the highest position

Patient position change is useful for observation. The principle is to move the region to be observed in the highest position, namely using the left lateral position for observing the right-side colon, the right lateral position for the left-side colon, and the left lateral position for the rectum. When the region to be observed is moved up, the colonic fluid and residue move to the bottom and the air moves to the top, allowing the lumen to be expanded, thereby facilitating observation.

4. Observe the inner sides of the bends carefully

Blind areas tend to occur in acute bends, which include the R-S, S-D, splenic flexure, the bend in the mid-transverse colon, the inner side of the hepatic flexure and the back side of Bauhin's valve. Observation while withdrawing the scope is often difficult in these regions. When observing each bend, it is recommended to push the scope slightly to apply it to the wall on the opposite side and observe the bend as if looking at it backwards. The scope tip can be retroflexed wherever possible.

5. Observe the sigmoid colon by re-inserting scope

After completing observation by withdrawing the scope as far as the rectum, insert the scope into the sigmoid colon again and observe it. At this time, it is a good idea to form a loop and stretch the intestinal tract to decrease the blind areas.

6. Use retroflexed observation in the vicinity of the anus

Surprisingly, the area in vicinity to the anus can often be hidden. Therefore, be sure to use the retroflexion technique in this region at the end of observation. To retroflex the scope tip, apply it to a wall near the second Houston valve, angulate it upward to the maximum and push in gently. Pulling the scope moves it towards the anal canal, while pushing it moves it away from the anal canal. To cancel the retroflexion, neutralize the angulation and pull the scope.

7. Use dyes as required

If any irregularity is detected during normal observation, spraying indigo carmine may lead to the discovery of an unexpected lesion. It is not recommended to regard dye spraying as a special examination technique; instead, it should be considered a routine tool for assisting examinations.

③ Always pay attention to superficial elevated type and depressed type lesions

Hiroshi Kashida

Finding inflammatory bowel disease, advanced colorectal carcinoma or protruded polyp is not that difficult except in certain blind areas. What is important is knowing how to detect superficial elevated type and depressed type lesions without missing them.

1. Viewing without noticing

Endoscopists who are not accustomed to seeing superficial elevated type or depressed type lesions, including beginners and Western doctors, do not notice such lesions even when they are shown on the monitor image. This may be because they do not have much experience with these types of lesions, and so have not acquired the pattern recognition or basically are not really looking for them. It is necessary to look at many pictures of these kinds of lesions in textbooks and lectures.

2. Pay attention to slight differences in color tone and gloss

In normal endoscopic images, superficial elevated type and depressed type lesions are characterized by slight reddening or discoloration, slight wall deformation, interruption of capillary network and spontaneous bleeding. Laterally spreading tumors (LSTs) can be quite large, with a diameter of several centimeters, but often escape detection because of their low height and color tone almost the same as the normal mucosa. The clue that makes discovery possible is a slight difference in gloss.

There are cases in which the lesion itself is not in view but only the surrounding white spots are visible. These can often be the clue to discovering a superficial elevated type or depressed type lesion, as well as an advanced carcinoma.

3. Insufflation does not always make lesions more noticeable

People tend to think that insufflating air can help increase the visibility of lesions during observation. This is of course important, but repetition of insufflation and deflation of air can also facilitate lesion detection by changing the view of observed area into frontal view, tangential-direction view, etc. A lesion can sometimes be found by noticing an area with poor movement during the repetition of insufflation and deflation.

In the case of a depressed type cancer, whether the depression depth is emphasized by deflation (which is referred to as air-induced deformation) serves for differentiation from an adenoma with pseudodepression as well as for prediction of cancer depth.

To reduce the discomfort of the patient, it is recommended to deflate air of each segment right after its observation is over during scope withdrawal.

4. Patient posture change is often useful

The basic patient posture for observing the rectum is the left lateral position and that for other regions is the supine position. It sometimes happens that what was visible during scope insertion cannot be found during withdrawal. In such a case, putting the patient back to the original position used during insertion often makes the suspected lesion visible again.

If a lesion detected during a barium enema study or previous colonoscopy cannot be found, try various patient postures. In addition, when a lesion is found, select the best posture for observing the total image of the lesion. When treating a lesion, the posture should also be changed to that most suitable for treatment.

5. Dye spraying is essential

Many endoscopists, including myself, routinely perform pit pattern diagnosis using magnifying endoscopy. Even for those who do not, dye spraying is indispensable. This is because dye spraying is extremely useful for clarifying the presence of a depression and its shape, and the range of an LST lesion. However, keep in mind that dye spraying is not a means of finding lesions; it is a means of confirming a lesion suspected in an ordinary view and examining it in detail. Relying on dye to detect lesions could result in paying less attention during ordinary observation.

④ How to avoid missing lesions in blind spots

Satoru Tamura

1. During insertion

Because successful scope insertion requires using as little air as possible, detailed observation is not possible during insertion. Nevertheless, since the condition of colon folds changes during insertion and withdrawal, lesions found during insertion can be lost to view during withdrawal. This does not pose a problem if the position of lesion can be identified accurately, but with the sigmoid colon, descending colon and transverse colon, it is necessary to check the tumor diameter and morphology of each lesion and determine whether follow-up is possible during insertion.

Since depressed-type lesions — even those as small as, or smaller than, 5 mm — require early treatment if they are of the depressed type, tattooing or clipping may be applied when required. Keep in mind that spending too much time on observation may make insertion to the cecum difficult.

2. During withdrawal

Observation in colonoscopy is performed mainly during withdrawal of the scope.

1) Changes on mucosal surfaces

Elevated lesions are usually not overlooked provided that they are within the field of view. However, since depressed or non-granular type laterally spreading tumors (LSTs) are not much different in color tone, they can easily be overlooked unless you are consciously keeping an eye out for them. It is essential to look for slight reddening, height irregularities on mucosal surfaces, and disappearance of visible vascular patterns.

2) Blind spots

Blind spots occur on bends and on the proximal sides of folds.

　　Cecum: Inner side of the lower lip of Bauhin's valve.

　　Ascending colon: Inner side of the hepatic flexure.

　　Transverse colon: Proximal sides of the central bend and splenic flexure.

　　Descending colon: Proximal side of the D-S junction.

　　Sigmoid colon: Entire region because of a large number of bends.

　　Rectum: Proximal side of the middle rectal valve of the rectum above the peritoneal reflection (Ra) and the posterior wall of the rectum below the peritoneal reflection (Rb).

　　The middle rectal valve is usually well developed so it tends to become a blind spot.

　　The posterior wall of Rb forms the boundary with the anal verge, and the scope often sneaks through it. This region should also be observed carefully by varying the amount of air, and retroflexing the scope's distal end is not always necessarily.

3. Varying the amount of air

To avoid missing lesions in blind spots, observe the folds by flipping them with the scope. However, since you will never have enough time for the procedure if you observe every fold in this way, it is important to insufflate and suction air to vary the lumen surfaces permanently in regions with many folds.

4. Easily missed lesions

1) Depressed lesions

Since a depressed carcinoma causes submucosal invasion when the diameter is 5 to 10 mm and becomes a carcinoma which indicate surgical intervention, when it is 10 mm or more, detecting the presence of lesions of around 5 mm diameters is important from a viewpoint of endoscopic diagnosis.

Unlike polyps, depressed tumors are not noticeably different in height or color tone from normal mucosa. This means you have to remember to keep an eye out for them during observation by keeping the scope in freely controllable status and by varying the amount of air.

In normal observation, the main finding that indicates a depressed tumor is a slight reddening, which is sometimes recognized as a discolored area. It is also important to observe the wall deformation in lateral images.

When a lesion is confirmed, spray some dye and observe the properties of the depressed surface and its marginal zone in detail to determine whether the lesion is of the depressed type or not and whether it is benign or malignant. It is also necessary to diagnose the invasion depth to determine whether or not to apply EMR. A depressed lesion under dye spraying shows its depressed surface, which is distinguishable from the spiny irregularities characteristic of the depressed area in the lesion of IIa + dep.

2) Non-granular type LSTs

LSTs are classified into granular and non-granular types. Non-granular type LSTs do not have a granular structure on the surface, and show virtually no difference in color tone from the mucosa, making their presence very difficult to diagnose. Clues that can help detect these lesions include wall deformation, disappearance of visible vascular patterns and irregularities on the mucosal surface.

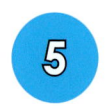

⑤ Tips on detection and diagnosis

Osamu Tsuruta, Hiroshi Kawano

1. Tips on detection

Detecting lesions accurately is essential in colonoscopy. As certain types of lesion are easy to miss, careful observation supported by knowledge of the findings that can be clues to the presence of a lesion is crucial.

1) Change in color tone

During observation of a mucosal surface in the long- or medium-distance view, you may see an isolated area that presents a different color tone from the surrounding mucosa. This finding can often lead to the detection of a superficial tumor. The color tone usually changes to reddish but can also look like discoloration, particularly in the presence of melanosis.

2) Change in visible vascular pattern

This change is usually confirmed after the change in color tone. Even when there is no change in color tone, the presence of a lesion can sometimes be detected from the difference between the visible vascular image and the surrounding normal mucosa. With tumorous lesions, the abnormality is usually indicated by the disappearance of the visible vascular pattern, but can also be indicated by differences in the pattern.

3) Thickening of folds

Superficial tumors whose color tone does not differ from the surrounding normal mucosa may be recognized by slight thickening of folds.

4) Presence of white spots

Lesions surrounded by white spots are frequently encountered. However, in a bend, it is sometimes impossible to find the lesion itself, even though white spots have been observed. Whenever white spots are observed, you should assume that a lesion exists nearby and examine the proximity closely.

5) Eliminating blind spots

a) Regulating the air amount

Basically, observation is performed by insufflating a fair amount of air to stretch the intestinal wall. However, by decreasing the amount of air when observing the oral side of a fold or bend, you may be able to bring the previously unobservable region into view.

b) Changing the patient's position

Changing the patient's position changes the contours of the intestinal tract, sometimes improving the view of a previously hard-to-view region. In addition, even when insufflating air fails to stretch the intestinal tract, the movement of air induced by position change may succeed in doing so.

c) Using forceps or other devices

If none of the above methods makes it possible to observe the oral side of a fold or bend, pushing the fold or intestinal tract aside mechanically using forceps or another device may make it possible to view the oral side.

d) Retroflexed observation

Though retroflexion is difficult in some regions, it is relatively easy in the ascending colon and rectum. Retroflexed observation is necessary whenever observation from the anal side seems insufficient.

2. Tips on diagnosis

If you encounter something that appears to be a lesion, perform qualitative and quantitative diagnoses.

1) Washing the lesion and surroundings

Since residue and mucus make it difficult to evaluate a lesion, the lesion and surrounding area need to be washed.

2) Presence of innominate grooves

If the suspected lesion has innominate grooves similar to those present on the surrounding normal mucosa, it is not hyperplasia or a tumorous lesion but the result of an inflammation or capillary dilatation. If, on the other hand, there are no innominate grooves, assume that the lesion is tumorous and proceed to more detailed observation.

3) Distant-view observation

To objectively identify the size and shape of a lesion, it should first be observed in the distant view. Observing the changes in the lesion morphology depending on the amount of air and the degree of tension in the surface of normal mucosa around the lesion in the overstretched status makes it possible to check the size of the lesion itself.

4) Observation from as many directions as possible

Try to collect as much information on the lesion surface without leaving a dead angle. A superficial tumor should also be observed from the lateral direction in order to view the height and depression depth objectively.

5) Close-up view observation

Recent scopes — even those without magnifying capability — are often capable of pit-pattern observation, enabling you to differentiate between a tumor and non-tumor. Observation of vascular patterns has also been demonstrated to be useful for qualitative and quantitative diagnoses. Although a magnifying scope is desirable, the close-up view obtained with an ordinary scope is also useful.

⑥ Tips on accurate qualitative diagnosis using standard colonoscopic observation

Shinji Tanaka

1. Discard preconceived ideas when screening

The most important thing when screening lesions is to discard the idea that "colon = polyp". Colonoscopy demands the same perspective and focus used to detect a 0-IIc early gastric carcinoma. It is important to understand this fact when screening superficial (particularly the 0-IIc type) lesions.

It is also important to increase and decrease the amount of air by repeating suction and insufflation during observation. Overstretching the colorectum not only makes it more difficult to observe regions that tend to have dead angles such as bends and the backsides of folds, but also interferes with the detection of superficial lesions. Try to keep the colorectum stretched at an optimum level to facilitate detection of air-induced deformations and changes in surface properties and colors of the lesions.

2. Tips on standard colonoscopic observation of a localized lesion

The most important thing to remember in standard colonoscopic observation of a localized lesion is to observe it from various angles (frontal and lateral images) with various air amounts, and from various distances — long-distance, medium-distance and close-up. Specific observation items include macroscopic classification, size, colors, surface properties (depression, erosion, surface irregularities, granules/nodules), fold concentrated/wrinkled images and peripheral hardening image.

The distant view captured with a relatively large amount of air provides an overall image of the lesion useful for identification and for detection of invasion findings from the images of hardening and wrinkling. Images captured with a small amount of air are useful for diagnoses of the air-induced deformation of tumor and the invasion depth based on the volume effect of the submucosal layer, while close-up images are indispensable for the diagnosis of microstructure on the lesion surface.

3. Observation using dye spraying

In observation with dye spraying, the key is to wash off mucus and stool liquid attached to the lesion surface with water. When using one of the latest videoscopes, you will be able to observe the innominate grooves just by eliminating the mucus.

In addition, spraying indigo carmine solution enables diagnosis of most large pit structures and also makes it possible to obtain other information such as histological atypia, the presence and properties of depressed areas, and the tumor growth pattern. On the other hand, if dye is sprayed without eliminating the mucus, the surface structure is unclear and observation conditions will deteriorate considerably.

4. Tips on washing the lesion

The tips on washing the lesion include: ① use lukewarm water instead of cool water (to prevent spasms); ② mix a small amount of Gascon® in the lukewarm water (to prevent bubble production); ③ target the margin instead of the lesion itself so that the lesion is washed by the flow from the margin (to prevent bleeding from lesion); ④ if washing the lesion directly with the spray, reduce the water pressure to prevent bleeding; ⑤ if attached mucus is hard to eliminate, use protease as required.

These purocedures are no trouble to perform. Simply prepare Gascon® solution and inject it directly from the scope's forceps channel using a syringe.

When using one of the latest videoscopes, do not use the same photo quality level as used with an old fiberoptic scope. Accurate qualitative diagnosis is not possible unless observation (photographing) is accurate enough to enable evaluation of findings.

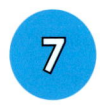

7. Important points to keep in mind during observation

Yusuke Saitoh

Important points
- The purpose of colonoscopy is not to reach the cecum, but to find lesions. Pay attention to the minute findings such as slight reddishness and discoloration, and use a dye spraying method when a lesion is suspected.
- In the right-side colon, make sure to observe the back side of haustra folds.
- To prevent the scope from suddenly slipping backwards in the transverse colon during scope withdrawal, keep the scope straight, repeat fine pushing and pulling (jiggling), and withdraw slowly.
- For observation from the left side of the transverse colon to the descending colon, use the right lateral position as required.
- Observe the rectum with retroflexed observation whenever possible.

The purpose of colonoscopy is not to reach the cecum but to find lesions. That means that observation is the most important aspect of the colonoscopic procedures. Maintain your concentration at all times during observation and pay full attention to minute findings such as slight reddishness or discoloration.

When you have even the slightest suspicion that a lesion is present, use a dye spraying method using 0.1% indigo carmine solution to determine whether or not one is present. Insufflate enough air to expand the lumen sufficiently for observation. After completing observation of the region, suction air until the lumen shrinks a little, then move on to the next region.

If a mucosa is suctioned, it will be observed as slight reddishness, which is hard to distinguish from a superficial tumor unless sprayed with dye. To prevent suctioning of the mucosa, the suction force should be set to a fairly low setting.

The points to note in each region are as described below.

To observe the extent from the cecum to the right side of the transverse colon, place the patient in the supine position or left lateral position. Pay special attention to the back side of the ileocecal valve in the cecum. In the right-side colon where haustras are prominent, the back sides of the haustras tend to be overlooked easily. Since the LSTs (laterally spreading tumors) that are frequently found in this region are often spread across the haustra folds, it is important to remember to check the back sides of haustras during observation. A common technique that I use is to rotate the scope counterclockwise along the mucosa in the lumen.

In the transverse colon, the scope often slips backward suddenly, making it necessary to move forward and back inside the colon several times. As a result, almost all endoscopists have had the experience of causing the patient unnecessary pain. To prevent the scope from suddenly slipping backwards in the transverse colon during scope withdrawal, it is recommended to keep the scope straight (in the shape of the number 7), repeat fine pushing and pulling (jiggling), and withdraw slowly.

Observation from the left side of the transverse colon to the descending colon is generally performed with the patient in the supine position with the left lumbar slightly elevated. If this does not expand the descending colon sufficiently, use the right lateral position.

For observation from the sigmoid colon to the rectum, use the left lateral position. If you were able to shorten the sigmoid colon during insertion, insufflate enough air during withdrawal to facilitate observation.

The incidence of the lesions is quite high in the rectum. Lesions immediately above the anal canal are often first discovered with retroflexed observation, so it is recommended to perform retroflexed observation in the rectum whenever possible. Retroflexed observation of the rectum can be performed relatively safely by angulating the scope up and to the left as far as it will go, then pushing the scope along Houston's valve. However, retroflexed observation in the rectum should be done cautiously with patients who have a small build, particularly elderly patients. Use a thin and/or pliant scope for retroflexed observation of these patients.

15. Retroflexed Observation in the Rectum

① Rectal observation is a must

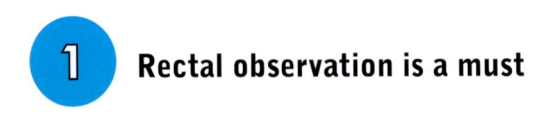

Hiroyuki Tsukagoshi

Retroflexed observation in the rectum, observation of the appendiceal orifice, and insertion into the terminal ileum should always be a part of any colonoscopic procedure. The techniques used are easy and risk-free.

1. Why retroflexed observation in the rectum is necessary

The lower rectum is the most important region observed in colonoscopy. Since advancement of carcinoma in this region is highly likely to result in the need for an artificial anus, it is preferable to treat it while it is an adenoma or an intramucosal cancer.

While the rate of detection of depressed early colon cancer in the colon has been increasing recently, the rate of detection in the lower rectum is low. The reason for this is not known. However, as the lower rectum is not difficult to observe, efforts should be made to increase detection in this region, as well.

To perform retroflexed observation, apply the scope's distal end perpendicularly against the rectal wall before the Houston valve, angulate the scope as far up as it will go, and push the scope to retroflex the distal end spontaneously. Although there is usually no resistance, if resistance is felt, the patient complains about pain, and you are a beginner, do not continue observation. Replace the scope with a slimmer one and retry.

The region in the rectum that is most difficult to observe is the posterior wall. When the scope enters from the anus, the region initially viewed in the front of the scope is the anterior wall. The posterior wall is recessed like a cave and often hidden from view.

Even when retroflexed observation is used in the rectum, the posterior wall is sometimes hidden behind the scope and hard to view. If the posterior wall cannot be properly observed, a digital rectal examination should also be performed. This will make it possible to check for anal canal carcinoma at the same time.

2. The key to mastering colonoscopy is the ileocecal valve insertion method

There is one thing I would like to say about insertion through the ileocecal valve. While difficult, insertion into the ileocecal valve provides ideal exercise for mastering colonoscopic insertion with a small amount of air.

When inserting the scope into the ileum through the ileocecal valve, suction air at a point slightly past the ileocecal valve, angulate the scope upward and pull it back, while keeping the tip in contact with the mucosa as if scraping off a thin layer of skin.

If the orientation and angle of the scope do not accurately correspond with the colon, you will not be able to insert it successfully. Manipulate the scope as slowly as possible. The image on the monitor becomes a close-up image. The series of maneuvers described above have much in common with the basic techniques used to insert the colonoscope into the colon.

② Observation without dead angles

Masao Ando

1. Observing the anterior wall during withdrawal

On completion of observation, put the patient in the left lateral position and check the region from the rectum (Rb) to the anus while withdrawing the scope. While doing this, deliberately vary the amount of air between the anterior and posterior walls, and compress the scope to avoid creating dead angles.

The anterior wall is usually easy to observe, but the posterior wall often has blind spots where observation is difficult because it runs in the tangential direction for a relatively long distance (a few centimeters). Examining this area carefully is the most important part of the retroflexed observation.

2. Retroflexed observation technique

To retroflex the scope in the rectum to place the scope shaft along the anterior wall and angulate it up toward the sacrum. At the same time, angulate it to the left by applying pressure with the tip of your left thumb.

When the scope is angulated to the maximum and pushed in slowly with the right hand, a frontal view of the posterior wall of Rb can be obtained. If a slim, pliant scope is used, this can be achieved with virtually no resistance. Do not use force if you do feel any resistance or if the patient complains about pain.

If a stiff scope with long distal-end rigid section is used, retroflexion inside the rectum may not be possible in some cases. If so, try another scope.

3. Observation method

After observing the entire posterior wall, rotate the scope toward the anterior wall to observe it. You should usually rotate the scope clockwise for this purpose, but you can also observe the anterior wall using counterclockwise rotation as required, provided that there is no resistance.

Simply retroflexing the scope may result in dead angles being created in the proximity of the anus or make it difficult to observe the status of internal hemorrhoids. To check these regions, keep the scope retroflexed, and slowly push it in and pull it back while regulating the amount of air (usually this means insufflating additional air).

After completing observation, cancel the retroflexion, check the inside of the rectum once more, then withdraw the scope while suctioning air. Deaeration can reduce the dead angles behind folds and on the posterior wall of Rb.

③ The purpose of retroflexed observation and some points to remember

Sumio Tsuda

Even when a scope with a wide field of view and excellent distal-end mobility is used, the area observable with the frontal view of a forward-viewing scope is limited. To avoid overlooking lesions when observing particularly difficult areas such as the rectum below the peritoneal reflection (Rb) and the back side of the Houston valve, the scope should be retroflexed.

1. Retroflexion method

The scope can be retroflexed by controlling the angulation knob with the left hand and manipulating the scope shaft with the right hand as appropriate, while taking care not to overstretch or injure the intestinal wall with the scope's distal end. The key points to remember are to manipulate the scope slowly and, while rotating the angulation knob, to push the scope shaft a little with the right hand when the scope shaft is about to contact the intestinal wall. Retroflexion can be canceled by exactly reversing the order of retroflexion procedure steps.

As you will need a sufficient space in the lumen in order to retroflex the scope, insufflate air to stretch the rectum before proceeding to retroflexion. Remember that each lumen is different and take this into account when insufflating.

Also note that the success of retroflexion can depend on the type of scope used. Obviously, a scope with a smaller distal-end bending section radius and narrower distal-end outer diameter is going to be more mobile and easier to manipulate in a lumen of the same size. If the scope is going to be retroflexed in a narrow lumen, be sure to select such a slim scope.

2. Retroflexed observation

After retroflexing the scope tip, perform retroflexed observation by pushing and pulling the scope, rotating the scope shaft in both directions and angulating the scope in the up, down, right and left directions. The bending angle can be as wide as 210° or so. In addition to scope manipulation, regulate the amount of air during observation. Retroflexion is also useful in endoscopic treatment. In cases where it is not possible to approach the lesion from the oral side, retroflexing the scope will make it possible to perform treatment successfully.

3. Danger of injury

Be very careful when retroflexing the scope if sufficient lumen width cannot be assured. Forced retroflexion presents a high potential of injuring the intestinal tract and causing serious complications.

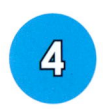

④ Do not take it easy during observation of the rectum

Hiroshi Kashida

1. Why so many lesions are missed in the rectum

In forward viewing, the mucosa of the lower rectum (Rb) is located behind the scope's distal end and cannot easily be brought into view. Consequently, lesions in this region tend to be overlooked (**Fig. 15-4-1**). Even advanced cancers are sometimes missed in this segment.

It is well known that LSTs occur frequently in the rectum. Because LSTs are large, they can often be in the field of view even if the scope is not retroflexed. Nevertheless, they still tend to be missed because their height and color tone do not differ substantially from normal mucosa.

2. Retroflex observation

The optimal position for the patient is the left lateral position. Since the lumen of the rectum is narrow compared to the stomach, retroflexing the scope all at once can be not only difficult, but also dangerous. Place the scope tip in the upper rectum (Ra) where the lumen is widest and angulate it slowly upward while pushing it little by little.

When the scope is fully angulated, rotate it axially with the right hand so that the inner side of the Rb is clearly visible. If the scope tip is too far from the anus, pull the scope slightly. Also adjust the left-right angulation and observe the whole area so that you do not miss any lesions. As the area behind the scope shaft tends to be hidden from view, be sure to observe from multiple angles using axial rotation and left-right angulation.

When a lesion is present in Rb and colostomy is indicated if it is subjected to surgery, it is important to measure the distance from the dentate line to the lesion. In such a case, the distance can often be measured more accurately in a retroflex view. In endoscopic treatment, retroflexion is required when incising or dissecting a large LST from the proximal side.

3. Precautions for retroflexion

During the retroflexion maneuver, the scope's distal end is directly pushed against to the mucosa until the scope is completely retroflexed. As a result, the image on the monitor often turns red, which means there is a risk of perforation. Discontinue retroflexion if strong resistance is felt or if the patient complains of severe pain.

It is a good idea to retroflex the scope in the widest part of the lumen. Narrow regions such as the Rs-S junction or the sigmoid colon should be avoided. Note that careless retroflexion may injure the mucosa or a lesion and hinder its observation.

4. Other techniques useful for observing the rectum

In my opinion, it is not necessary to retroflex the scope in all cases. There are other ways to ensure that lesions are not missed even if the scope is not retroflexed. With forward viewing, the mucosa in the Rb increasingly disappears behind the scope as the amount of insufflation increases. On the contrary, the mucosa approaches to the scope and enters into the field of view when air is suctioned sufficiently (**Fig. 15-4-1**).

It is not wise to assume that retroflexed observation will assure that no lesions are missed. Special care is required for the mucosa inside the anal canal because it is often hidden from the view of the scope when it is retroflexed (**Fig. 15-4-1**). It is therefore important to observe this region carefully after suctioning air in forward viewing, by moving the scope back and forth several times.

Finally, since many LSTs may be present in the rectum, pay attention to small differences in the color tone of the mucosa and use dye spraying as required.

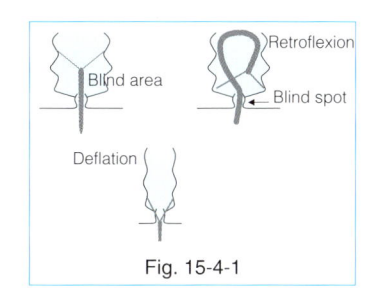

Fig. 15-4-1

⑤ Eliminating blind spots in rectal observation by retroflexing the scope

Osamu Tsuruta, Hiroshi Kawano

As well as bending sharply backwards in the lower part (Rb), the rectum has three Houston valves which result in blind spots on the oral side of the Houston valve, the posterior wall of Rb and the vicinity of the dentate line when observing exclusively from the anal side using a forward-viewing scope.

To eliminate these blind spots, it is absolutely necessary to retroflex the scope. The following describes the techniques used for scope retroflexion and observation in the rectum.

1. Retroflexion in the rectum (Fig. 15-5-1)

1) Stretch the rectum. (Fig. 15-5-1a)
Retroflexion is easier when there is plenty of space to maneuver the scope. Put the patient in the left lateral position and insufflate sufficient air to stretch the rectum.

2) Decide where you are going to retroflex the scope. (Fig. 15-5-1b)
It is easier to retroflex the scope by pressing the distal end against the intestinal wall, rather than by manipulating the scope in the space inside the lumen. Confirm the position of the Houston valve (usually the middle Houston valve) projecting into the inner cavity.

3) Angulate the scope upward. (Fig. 15-5-1c)
While approaching the Houston valve, slowly angulate the scope upward.

4) Add leftward angulation. (Fig. 15-5-1d)
Once the scope has neared the limit of upward angulation, start angulating it to the left, as well. Push the scope a little; the scope shaft will come in the view, confirming the retroflexion of the distal end. Operate both the upward and leftward angulation knobs with the left thumb. The reason leftward angulation is added is that it can increase the bending

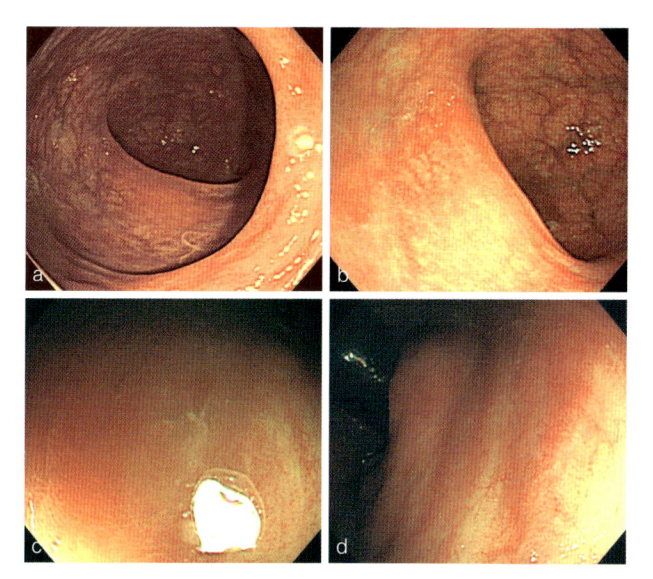

Fig. 15-5-1 Intrarectal retroflexion procedure
a) Stretch the rectum sufficiently.
b) Decide where the scope is to be retroflexed.
c) Angulate the scope slowly upward while approaching the Houston valve.
d) Add leftward angulation to the upward angulation and push the scope a little; the scope shaft will come into view, confirming retroflexion of the distal end.

angle of the scope's distal end more than upward angulation alone.

2. Retroflexed observation (Fig. 15-5-2)

1) Reserve a field of view in which the rectum can be observed circumferentially.

After confirming retroflexion, adjust the field of view so that the rectum can be observed circumferentially by angulating, rotating, pushing and pulling the scope. Return the scope's bending section to the neutral position for observation of the rectum.

2) Observe the oral side of the Houston valve. (Fig. 15-5-2a)

After pushing in the scope until no resistance is felt, pull the scope and observe the oral side of the Houston valve. During observation, adjust the

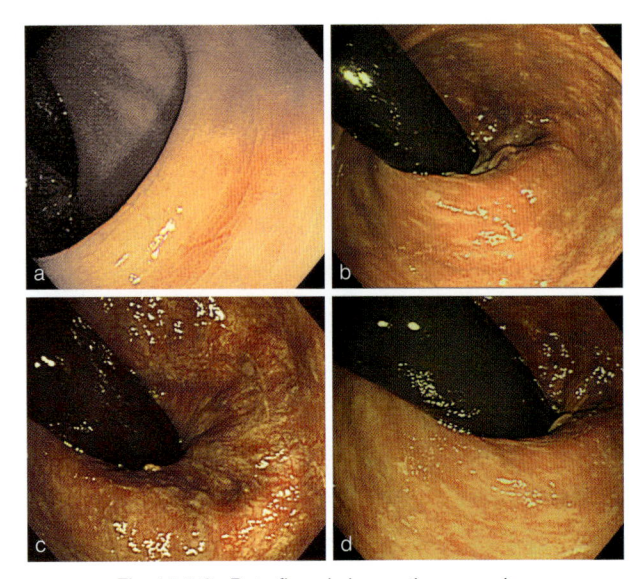

Fig. 15-5-2 Retroflexed observation procedure
a) Observe the oral side of the Houston valve.
b) Observe the Rb posterior wall.
c), d) Observe the vicinity of the dentate line.

field of view by angulating and rotating the scope.

3) Observe the Rb posterior wall. (Fig. 15-5-2b)

Pull the scope back some more and thoroughly observe the posterior wall of Rb.

4) Observe the vicinity of the dentate line. (Fig. 15-5-2c, d)

For the most part, circumferential observation is possible by rotating the scope. Increasing the amount of air even makes it possible to observe part of the anal canal.

16. Dye Spraying

1 Dye spraying, safety of dyes

Satoru Tamura

When a lesion is found or suspected in normal observation, dye is sprayed in the region and pit pattern observation is performed using a magnifying videoscope. The detected lesion is first washed with water containing antifoaming agent to remove mucus on the surface, taking care not to use too much pressure in order to prevent bleeding from the surface. It is best to use lukewarm water as cold water may induce peristalsis.

After washing the lesion, spray it with 0.2% indigo carmine solution from the forceps channel (inject 4 to 5 ml of solution in a 20-ml syringe and push the solution with about 15 ml of air to spray the solution on the surface). This technique is a contrast method.

First, the normal chromoendoscopic image is observed in detail to check the lesion boundary, surface height irregularities and the presence of demarcated depressed areas.

Next, increase the magnification and approach the scope's distal end to observe the pit pattern. (Since this is a contrast method, the pit opening will appear as an area where dye has pooled.)

Chromoendoscopy using indigo carmine and pit pattern diagnosis is sufficient for ordinary lesions. However, when a carcinoma is suspected, the next step is to perform dye staining for accurate qualitative diagnosis and invasion depth diagnosis.

After washing the lesion with water again, dye only the lesion area with about 0.05% solution of methylrosanilinium chloride (gentian violet, crystal violet, pyoktanin blue) using an injection tube, and observe the pit pattern. (Since this technique is a staining method, the pit opening is observed as a non-stained area).

Crystal violet (pyoktanin) has long been used in the form of water solutions or ointments in dermatology or as a gargle for oral candida, and a 1/20 solution is frequently used in targeted staining. In addition, for a variety of reasons including the quick turnover of mucosal cells in the colon, the likelihood that the lesion will be resected on the same day or within a few days, and the absence of any reports on disorder induced locally or in other organs due to its use, this dye is considered completely safe when used in local staining.

② Reasons for dye spraying and how to do it

Sumio Tsuda

Colorectal diseases are diagnosed with standard colonoscopy as well as chromoendoscopy, an invaluable diagnostic modality used for finding, qualitative diagnosis and invasion depth diagnosis of tumors and tumorous lesions. Though not always necessary with inflammatory bowel diseases, it can help facilitate clear observation of ulcers, erosion and aphtha, as well as clarifying the properties of the mucosa surrounding them.

1. Chromoendoscopy in the colon and rectum
This includes a staining method using methylene blue, etc. and a contrast method using indigo carmine. For ordinary colonoscopy, a simplified contrast method using 0.1% indigo carmine solution is adequate.

2. Dye-spraying procedure
Before spraying the dye, wash away the bubbles, mucus and stool attached to the lesion and the surrounding area. The dye spraying tube is not used because it may cause the lesion to start bleeding. Fill a 20-ml syringe with dye solution and spray it directly from the scope's forceps channel. Spray the dye slowly and thoroughly, being sure to evenly cover the lesion and the area around it.

After spraying the dye, suction off any excess dye. Be careful not to injure the lesion or the surrounding mucosa. Even if the initial washing seemed sufficient, some mucus may still remain on and around the lesion. In this case, repeat washing and dye spraying until the mucus is eliminated completely.

3. Points to heed when spraying the dye

Regardless of whether it is a tumor, a tumorous lesion, or inflammatory bowel disease, do not spray only the conspicuous lesion. Since the surrounding conditions have to be taken into consideration when making a diagnosis, it is essential to spray the dye evenly over the entire observable range.

③ Contrasting technique

Osamu Tsuruta, Hiroshi Kawano

The two primary methods of dye spraying are the contrast method and the staining method. Here, we will discuss the contrast method. This method clarifies the height irregularity of a lesion and facilitates identification of the range and surface properties including its shape and whether or not a depression is present.

1. Washing the lesion and surrounding area

Mucus and other residue on and around the lesion make it more difficult to determine the lesion's properties. Even when it appears as if there is no mucus left under normal observation, a large amount of mucus is sometimes discovered after dye spraying. Therefore, the site should be thoroughly washed before dye spraying. While washing the target area, be careful not to use too much pressure when applying the washing fluid as this could cause the lesion to start bleeding. Also do not use cold fluid as this could stimulate peristalsis of the intestinal tract. We use a syringe filled with lukewarm water in which a small amount of defoaming agent has been mixed and inject the solution through the biopsy port.

2. Dye spraying

1) Type and concentration of dye

In most cases, use a 0.1% indigo carmine solution (prepared by solving 20 mg/5 ml/A in 15 ml of lukewarm water). To avoid inducing peristalsis, do not use a cold solution.

2) Spraying method

One way of spraying dye is to inject the solution directly from the biopsy port; another is to use a washing tube. The first technique makes it easier to spray dye across a wider area, but precise adjustment is difficult and a large amount of dye has to be used. The second method is trickier to execute, but facilitates more precise control and does not require as much dye.

3) Sprayed area, injection rate

a) Spraying the lesion

Since spraying with too much pressure may induce bleeding from the lesion, the dye should be sprayed slowly if a washing tube is used — almost as if letting it drip onto the surface. Using a washing tube to spray dye is a good idea when you need to pool dye solution in the depressed region or to adjust the surface coverage. It is also convenient if you have to repeat the operation, as you leave the tube inside the scope. When pooling or moving the dye, it is recommended to change the patient position.

b) Spraying around the lesion

To diagnose the invasion depth of a carcinoma, it is necessary to check the degree of creasing around the lesion (stretching failure). To do this, spray the dye across a wide area around the lesion and observe it from a distance. This makes it possible to clearly observe even minor findings. The dye can be also sprayed with a fair amount of pressure because the area around the lesion does not bleed easily.

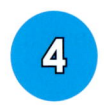

4 Contrast method and staining method

Masahiro Igarashi

There are two methods used in chromoendoscopy: the contrast method and the staining method.

1. Contrast method

Widely used in typical colonoscopic examinations, the contrast method is performed by spraying indigo carmine solution. The concentration can be selected as desired by each endoscopist, but we usually use the range between 0.5 and 1.0%. Indigo carmine spraying is excellent for screening of flat and depressed type tumorous lesions, as well as for detailed observation of the surface properties of tumorous and elevated lesions. It is useful for detailed diagnosis of inflammatory mucosa of inflammatory bowel diseases and is also used in combination with magnifying endoscopy for pit pattern diagnosis.

Indigo carmine can be sprayed using either a spraying cannula or directly via a syringe in the scope's biopsy port. Since indigo carmine can be washed away with water, it can be used repeatedly.

2. Staining method

Used primarily in magnifying endoscopic diagnoses, the staining method uses crystal violet or methylene blue dye. The most commonly used crystal violet concentration is 0.05%.

After spraying, it is necessary to wait for 2 or 3 minutes before starting observation. Moreover, since this technique stains the cells, the dye cannot be washed off. This means that if the dye is sprayed across a wide area, it will stain the entire intestinal tract, making subsequent observation difficult. In addition, as the dye is absorbed by cells, the stained area needs to be minimized from a safety standpoint. The key point is to stain the cells as if dropping the solution from an injection cannula or a dedicated cannula.

3. Appropriate applications for each method

In general, the usages of the contrast method and the staining method are divided as described below.

1) Contrast method

This is useful in screening of tumorous diseases, as well as flat or depressed type lesions. In normal observation, flat lesions are usually distinguished by a reddish appearance. Spraying indigo carmine can make changes in color tone easier see, occasionally revealing an unanticipated lesion. I keep indigo carmine handy during every procedure so that it can be sprayed immediately whenever necessary.

  Observation of inflammatory diseases: This technique is also useful in observation of inflammatory diseases as well as tumors. I normally use this technique together with a magnifying scope when searching for dysplasia of ulcerative colitis. It is especially useful for discerning mucosal patterns that differ from the surrounding mucosa.

2) Staining method

The staining method is used for pit pattern diagnosis in combination with magnifying endoscopy. If mucus has been completely removed and cells have been properly dyed, subsequent observation can be of high diagnostic value. The staining method is also useful in tissue diagnosis and invasion depth diagnosis of early carcinoma.

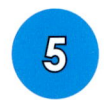

⑤ Tips on dye spraying and observation

Hiro-o Yamano

The chromoendoscopy consists of spraying a dye solution on the mucosa of the gastrointestinal tract. It is used to diagnose the extent and properties of lesion that are hard to identify with ordinary endoscopy.

In general, the dye spraying technique can be classified into the contrast method, staining method (in the narrow meaning of term) and reaction method depending on the characteristics of dyes used. The mainstreams of dye spraying technique in the colon and rectum are the contrast method using indigo carmine and the staining method using crystal violet or methylene blue.

1. Contrast method

Since ordinary endoscopy is not binocular, it has a difficulty in distinguishing fine undulation and shows it more planar than actually. This disadvantage makes it difficult to find lesions having same color tones as the surroundings.

This method is an application of the phenomenon of pooling of solutions of dye, such as indigo carmine, on a depressed micro-surface. It can enhance the surface irregularities on the membrane of the gastrointestinal tract, so it can be applied to observation of innominate grooves, detection of minute lesions, diagnosis of properties and determination of the extent of lesion.

Besides, the magnifying scope is capable of observing the morphology of crypt openings (so-called pit patterns). In our department, 0.2% indigo carmine solution (double solution of ready-made product) is used by adding a very small amount of Gascon® (2% dimethylpolysiloxane solution) for preventing foaming during spraying.

2. Staining method

This method dyes tissues *in vivo* by means of penetration of methylene blue or crystal violet, and is used in observation of the morphology of pit patterns. While the indigo carmine enables the observation of pits by pooling of the dye in them, the staining method stains the epithelium around the pits so the pits are observed by the absence of dye. As a result, the image obtained with this technique has the same relationship as the "negative and positive films in photography" with respect to the image obtained with the contrasting technique.

When the latest high-resolution magnifying scope is used, the pit pattern can be observed with similar clearness to the stereomicroscopic image. Nevertheless, this method also has some disadvantages, such as the difficulty in recognizing the fine undulation of the lesion and the overall darkness of the image because the dye also stains the mucosa around the lesion.

In our department, the observation based on the indigo carmine spraying is given the first priority while the staining method is used in detailed investigation by pinpoint staining using the dedicated spraying tube.

The tip on improving the diagnostic capabilities of dye-spraying examination is to wash away the mucus thoroughly, as far as the lesion does not bleed, before spraying the dye. For the observation condition, the tip on the contrast method is to observe the lesion immediately after dye spraying and that of the staining method is to start observation after leaving a certain period (1 to 2 min.) after dye spraying.

⑥ How to wash lesions and spray dyes

Shinji Tanaka

1. First, wash away mucus and stool liquid attached to the surface of the lesion

Whether the contrast method with indigo carmine or the staining method with crystal violet is used, always wash off any mucus and stool liquid on the lesion surface with water.

If you are using the latest videoscope, simply eliminating mucus allows the innominate grooves to be observed, while spraying indigo carmine solution allows the structures of large pits to be diagnosed, as well as providing information on the degree of histological atypia, the presence/properties of depressed areas, the tumor growth pattern, etc.

If there is still mucus on the lesion when dye is sprayed, the surface structure often becomes unclear and the observation conditions deteriorate even further.

2. Tips on washing the lesion

① Use lukewarm water instead of cool water (to prevent spasms).
② Mix a small amount of Gascon® in the lukewarm water (to prevent bubble production).
③ Target the perimeter instead of the lesion itself so that the lesion is washed by the flow from the perimeter (to prevent bleeding from lesion).
④ If spraying the lesion directly, reduce the water pressure to prevent bleeding.
⑤ If attached mucus is hard to eliminate, use protease as required.
These procedures can be performed easily by preparing Gascon® solution and injecting it directly from the scope's forceps channel using a syringe.

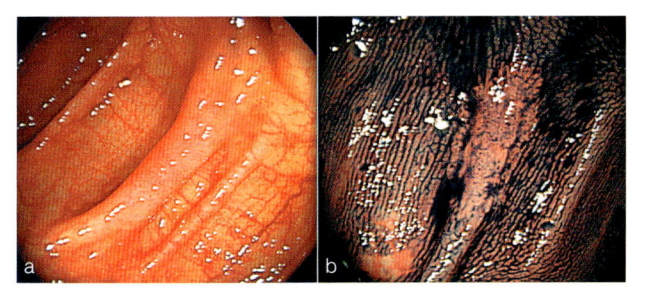

253

Fig. 16-6-1
a) With the standard colonoscopic observation image, only thick folds without any visible vascular pattern can be seen and it is impossible to distinguish between a tumor and inflammation.
b) After thoroughly washing the lesion and spraying it with indigo carmine, this is diagnosed as the lesion is a superficial tumor without the innominate grooves.

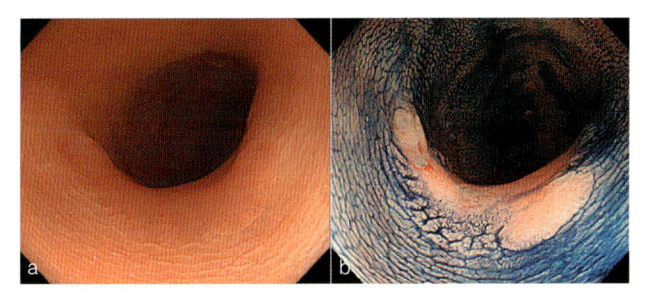

Fig. 16-6-2
a) Even in a normal observation image, innominate grooves around the tumor can be seen after it has been thoroughly washed.
b) The image obtained after indigo carmine dye spraying shows that a little bleeding has been produced by the high spraying pressure. To prevent such bleeding, it is not only necessary to regulate the spraying pressure, but also to be careful not to spray the lesion directly, but to spray the surrounding area so that the dye solution flows onto the lesion. That means that rather than using the spraying tube, insert a syringe directly into the forceps channel and inject indigo carmine.

3. Contrast method using indigo carmine

If the contrast method using indigo carmine is applied for tumor pit pattern diagnosis with magnifying endoscopy, it is recommended to spray a high-concentration solution. As with lesion washing, spraying the solution with too much pressure may cause bleeding so the spraying pressure should be regulated properly. When mucus is attached firmly to the lesion, using a low-concentration solution may enable clearer chromoendoscopic observation.

4. Staining method using crystal violet

The key to using crystal violet is to try to avoid staining the normal mucosa outside the tumorous lesion. If unnecessary areas are stained, the image will be dark like colonoscopic observation in tarry stool. When staining a broad area, the solution should be diluted considerably.

If the lesion is excessively stained, observation becomes difficult. How much staining occurs depends not just on the concentration of the solution, but also on the staining time and the characteristics of each lesion. It is recommended to perform the initial staining with a more diluted concentration and repeat staining as required.

Index

α, γ
α-loop 77, 78, 80, 82, 85, 87, 162, 164, 206
γ-loop 33, 105, 111, 112, 115, 120, 165, 172

A
abdominal palpation 43
adhesion 148, 150, 152, 154, 156, 158, 176, 178, 182, 198, 207
air amount 2, 4, 6, 8, 10, 12, 41, 69, 74, 123, 150, 152, 160, 189, 198, 217, 221, 224, 231, 232, 235
  regulating— 221
  varying— 217
air-induced deformation 215, 225
anal canal 58, 227, 231, 237, 240
  passing through— 59
anterior wall 93, 232
anus 48, 52, 58, 213, 232
  insertion into— 58
  observation of—and proximity 58
appendix orifice 142
ascending colon 124, 126, 128, 130, 132, 136, 138, 161, 212, 217

B
bend(bending section of intestinal tract) 2, 4, 8, 12, 56, 93, 124, 138, 141, 210, 213

blind spot 221, 238
bloody stool 176

C
cecum 138, 140, 142, 144, 146
cholecystectomy 151, 155
chromoendoscopy 242, 244, 248, 250
clinical histories 190
clockwise rotation 64
close-up view observation 222
colectomy 151
colic teniae 94
collapsed status of colon 10
color tone 214, 216, 220, 236, 249, 250
compound loop 82, 83
contrast method 242, 244, 246, 248, 250, 252, 254
counterclockwise rotation 64
crystal violet 242, 248, 250, 252, 254

D
dead angle 222, 224, 232
degassing 205
depressed type lesion 214, 216, 230, 247, 248, 250, 252
depression 192, 215, 242, 246
digital rectal examination 52, 58, 230
distant-view observation 222
dolichocolon 160, 162, 164, 166, 170
dolichosigmoid 163, 164, 166, 170

dolichotransversum   161, 165, 171
double loop   73, 166
dye spraying   212, 215, 218, 225,
   226, 237, 242, 244, 246,
   248, 250, 252

E
elderly patients   176, 182, 186,
   188, 190, 192, 200, 227
emergency colonoscopy   177
endoscope position detection
   system(UPD)   48, 163
erosion   224, 244

F
fold changes   216
fold concentrated/wrinkled image
   150, 160, 224
forceps   221

G
granules   224
gynecological cancer   150
gynecological surgery   152, 154, 158

H
hand pressure   16, 18, 20, 22, 24,
   28, 32, 130, 152, 174
hemorrhoid   43, 48, 52, 54, 58
hepatic flexure   13, 21, 30, 111,
   112, 114, 116, 119, 122,
   124, 126, 128, 130, 132,
   149, 155
hooking the fold   64, 72, 86, 105,
   114, 160

I
ideal reaching distances   122
ileocecal orifice   140
ileocecal valve   231

indigo carmine solution   213, 225,
   226, 242, 244, 246, 248,
   250, 252
inflammatory diseases   245, 248, 249
innominate grooves   221, 253
irregularities on the mucosal surface
   216, 218, 224, 250

L
large loop   167
laterally spreading tumor(LST)
   211, 214, 216, 218, 227, 236
left hand   8
lesion screening   224
long transverse colon   112
loop
   —in transverse colon   178
   α-—   77, 78, 80, 82, 85,
      87, 162, 164, 206
   γ-—   33, 105, 111, 112,
      115, 120, 165, 172
   double —   73, 166
   large —   167
   M-shaped —   164
   N-shaped —   67
lower rectum(Rb)   48, 56, 58, 62,
   217, 232, 234, 236, 238, 240
lubricant   50

M
macroscopic classification   224
magnifying observation   143, 215,
   248, 251
magnifying scope   48, 242, 248, 250
medication histories   190
melena   179
mesenteries   148
methylene blue   244, 248, 250, 251
mid-transverse colon   13, 112, 165
M-shaped loop   164

N
nodules 224
non-push technique 84
N-shaped loop 67

O
obesity 174
observation method 210, 232

P
pain 67
paradoxical movement 111, 114, 118, 128, 156
pattern A 78
pattern B 78
pattern C 79
pelvic radiation 176
perforation 43, 57, 149, 151, 157, 161, 170, 177, 184, 188, 196, 198, 200, 202, 204, 206, 208, 237
　checking — 205
peripheral hardening image 224
pit pattern 215, 222, 225, 242, 248, 250, 252, 254
polyp retrieval 45
position change 2, 5, 16, 18, 20, 22, 24, 28, 66, 92, 102, 104, 127, 128, 130, 132, 153, 174, 205, 221
　—impossible 178
post-cholecystectomy cases 151, 155
post-colectomy cases 151
posterior wall 232
post-gastrectomy cases 151, 154
postoperative adhesion 148, 156, 158, 207
premedication 9, 183, 193
pre-procedure interview 158
press & pass 19

pull-back 70, 89, 110, 113, 117, 119, 133, 136, 141, 144, 171, 189, 201
push technique 84, 158, 161, 174

Q
qualitative/quantitative diagnosis 224, 242, 244

R
radiation induced colitis 176
reciprocatory observation 210
rectal observation 230, 238
rectosigmoid colon(Rs) 16, 18, 56, 64, 78
respiratory assistance 130
retroflexed observation 19, 212, 221
　—in rectum 213, 226, 227, 230, 232, 234, 236, 237, 238
reverse α-loop 80
right-turn shortening 80, 83, 85, 161
Rs-S junction 44, 45, 53, 59, 62, 64, 66, 68, 70, 72, 74, 82

S
sagging 19, 119, 122, 133
　prevention of — 19, 23, 30, 36, 124, 129
scope selection 20, 48, 150, 153, 157, 176, 192
SD junction 32, 39, 76, 78, 80, 82, 84, 86, 88, 170, 206
shortening techniques 82, 183
sigmoid colon 76, 78, 82, 84, 86, 148, 160, 162, 178, 213
　—shortening technique 82, 86, 96, 162

—stretching technique 82
—volvulus 178, 179
sigmoid diverticula 176, 206
slalom technique 51, 122, 165
sliding tube 11, 36, 38, 39, 40, 42, 44, 50, 95, 131, 166, 168, 178
slight reddening 214
slit-like bending section 57
spastic colon 9
splenic flexure 20, 33, 85, 92, 93, 94, 96, 97, 98, 100, 101, 102, 104, 105, 110, 118, 154, 162, 163, 177
S-point 23, 131
staining method 242, 246, 248, 250, 252, 254
S-top 10, 12, 13, 45, 49, 51, 66, 87, 150, 164
straightening and shortening method 86
straightening of scope 76, 100, 116, 146
stretching techniques 82
superficial depressed type 214
superficial elevated type 214
surface irregularities 224, 250
surface properties 224, 246, 248

T
terminal ileum 136, 138, 140, 142, 144
—insertion 136
thin patient 115, 193

thin women 50, 176
three dimensional anatomy 62
T-point 23, 131
transparent hood 158
transverse colon 17, 18, 23, 30, 33, 92, 108, 110, 112, 114, 116, 118, 148, 161, 165, 171, 178, 208, 227
—loops 178
mid-— 13, 112, 165
passage of— 114
twisted intestinal tract 203

U
unnecessary scope manipulation 196
UPD(endoscope position detection system), 48, 163

V
Variable Stiffness scope 30, 38, 48, 95, 156
varying amount of air 217
visible vascular pattern 216, 218, 220, 253
disappearance of— 218
vital signs 186

W
wall deformation 214, 218
washing of lesion 221, 225, 242, 246, 252
white spots 214, 220
wrinkled fold 150, 160, 224